A BUTTERFLY
LANDED AN EAGLE

EDITION TWO

Twelve Years After *A Butterfly Landed An Eagle,*
And Eight Years After The Sequel *Eagles On The Highway:*
Now, Further Along This Highway (Of Life And For Life)...

D. ELIZABETH LAINE

Publisher: Inspiring Publishers,
P.O. Box 159, Calwell, ACT Australia 2905
Email: publishaspg@gmail.com
http://www.inspiringpublishers.com

A catalogue record for this book is available from the National Library of Australia

National Library of Australia The Prepublication Data Service

Author: D. Elizabeth Laine
Title: A Butterfly Landed an Eagle
Genre: Non-fiction

Print ISBN: 978-1-922792-75-4
Hardcover ISBN: 978-1-922920-14-0

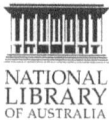

ABOUT THE AUTHOR

Elizabeth (Liz) Laine wrote *A Butterfly Landed An Eagle*. **D.** Elizabeth Laine, wrote the sequel, *Eagles On The Highway* (of life and for life). The initial (D) was added to distinguish her, from an English author, with the same name. Emphasis on **'I and N'** in La**i**ne, has been added, to represent, her mostly "North Indian" heritage. It has been added for the second edition, of *A Butterfly Landed An Eagle*.

The sequel proposed an, "Optimistic, Holistic (Body, Mind and Spirit), psycho-spiritual, model" for everyone, to optimistically, rebuild and mature, to deal with negativity (also strongholds) and "Bad things" of life (bad family legacies included). She applies her own theories, to her family legacies, as an example, to show, how best to deal with, bad things, once they have happened i.e. to overcome (in sequel) or manage them.

In the second edition of *A Butterfly Landed An Eagle*, she rewrites the book, to address the twelve years, since the first book was published, and eight since the sequel. Elizabeth, a retired Nurse, still resides in country WA, Australia with her husband Don, a retired Motor Mechanic. As a retired nurse, she is compelled to acknowledge, even with the best of intentions, theories are subject to choices, policy and process.

FORWARD

The first book (now out of print) and second edition, use an insect metaphor (for the 25,000 hours of childhood and cultural tape), to depict a pretty, fifteen year old, "Half Caste/Half Indian/Anglo-Indian" (represented by the first butterfly on the cover, one wing of an Indian flag and the other of an Irish kilt, for the 15 Irish clans in her DNA) migrant, which was actually more, "Asian-European" (new label for this chapter, under 'Family Of Origin' a course done), than 'Eurasian', or Pan-European, from the *Ancestry DNA*, done after both books were published. The next, "Butterfly" on the cover, with wings of an Australian flag, is for, Australian Citizenship, now in it's half century. The "Butterfly" was a derogatory term, once used by the mentally ill doctor (late first husband). The "Asian" part was mostly, "North Indian", like the childhood.

"Coming to Australia", was never about a, "Better Life", but, to 'Improve the bloodlines and merge back white' for the patriarch. Ironically, while the race was improved in six (so far) great grandchildren, the bloodline ended with the patriarch's death. Ancestry DNA uncovered English cousins, who didn't want to know their Indian counterpart (in Australia). Coming to Australia, put paid the dream, of becoming a doctor, so "Nursing chose me". At thirty nine, after an interview (one in twenty), to do medicine, as a mature age student (seventeen places), failed, the nursing degree, and a post-graduate Diploma in Orthopaedic nursing, was achieved by forty.

However, the university degrees from Curtin and Edith Cowan, didn't stem the derogatory terms, used by the family patriarch, or stop him comparing his two daughters, even when both sported degrees. Marrying a, "white" doctor to be, "accepted" didn't, "do it" either, so much for the romantic notions from *Barbara Cartland Novels* read as a teenager. Like the song, it was only ever *Imitation Love*. As a positive, both degrees, sit on file, as a permanent testament, to above average intelligence. "Lizzy girl" was not just a, "pretty dumb" nurse, or "Air-head" after all. So the Indian High School Certificate (at just 15) that was considered, only fourth year high, in Australia (Medicine required a Fifth year High School Certificate), did count! I know, I would've made, a good doctor.

Mental illness kept secret by the grooms side of the family, unchecked by parents of the bride, because, 'White was Right', led to chaos, dysfunctions and disorder. Four children, aged between one and seven, had to also deal with an absent dad as a, "Dr. M.D" (the initials also stood for Manic Depression). "Dr. Jekyll, Heckle and Hyde" from the cartoon, for a real, manic and depressed dad, now also depicts the 'Alter-egos', of the Schizophrenia part, of the renamed 'Schizo-Affective Disorder'. Diagnosed, or unknowingly misdiagnosed, with Bipolar II Disorder, probably accounted for, the 'Accidental' (coined in the sequel) suicide of a doctor, and possibly, also his maternal grandmother.

It made for, "The beginning of the end", not only for the marriage, but, coincided with the end of a nursing career, along with the death of romantic notions, from love story novels. Collateral damage, and general destruction of all relationships (friends and primary family included), are addressed by/as Eagles, further along the highway. The next generation lost their maternal grandmother. While sole custody was impossible, in past Bipolar Disorder cases, sole custody was granted in the Schizo-Affective disorder case, of the youngest offspring's, only child. Three, older, offspring, managed to complete university degrees, have careers, marriages and families (six as far as is known). The Mental Health System, has also undergone a renaissance, with a lot more emphasis, on social issues, by 'Case co-ordinators', working with guardians and the family in, "Teams", to support the mentally ill person, limited by choices, policy and process.

Chapter eight, now includes content, from the previous chapter nine "Growing fast tracked", as the Eagle has grown past this stage, over the ensuing twelve years, and is eight years, further along the highway (of life and for life). Edition two, is a re-write, to reflect the eight years since the sequel, *Eagles On The Highway* (now a reference in this edition) and 12 years since the first book, *A Butterfly Landed An Eagle*, were published (now out of print).

There have been more, "Weddings, Marriages, Divorces, Funerals, Deaths (one suicide and one unexpected) and Births" (now Chapter Nine). Some weddings were attended, but, not all marriages. While there were deaths in the family, not all funerals were attended. The births of all nine grandchildren (of both Eagles) have been recorded. Thanks to one remarriage, a, 'Secret lie', (that some liars took to their graves), was unearthed, further along the "Highway". Eagles no longer attend church, so "Churchianity; a new religion", has been deleted.

As both families of origin are deceased, family matters no longer mattered. Only legacies are left. "Family Matters", has been replaced, with the last, or tenth chapter, of (not the best way to apply a theory, proposed in the sequel, but), doing the best possible, to manage it, and then letting go i.e. "Damage Control and Letting Go" (and not only behind their backs, as in the sequel). There is no alternative, when dealing with 'Schizo-Affective Disorder' (a totally different 'kettle of fish'), as opposed to Manic Depression and/or Bipolar II . It re-defined the "Personality Disorder" for a grandfather, and the suicide of a father. In reflection, Schizophrenia had been a part of the disorder, right from the start, but, only discovered for both fathers, after their deaths.

The theory proposed in the sequel, is applicable, as an example. The legacies of lies and mental illness, left a majority 'People of the lie' (from *The Road Less Travelled* by the late psychiatrist, Dr. M. S. Peck, a reference in my sequel and in this edition), i.e.

people of lies (also liars) and mental illness (of primary family left). The battle rages, further along the 'Highway' (pro-life) also the *Road Less Travelled,* to do the best possible, 'Responsible To' (*Boundaries Course* and *Boundaries* by Doctors Cloud and Townsend), support the youngest daughter, who inherited the mental health legacy (limited by her rights as an adult, supporting her team, as part of the solution (with knowledge comes power), in 'Just Love' (coined in the sequel), before 'Letting Go".

The Eagle took her own advice, to holistically manage the "Body beating" (from the ongoing stress) *When Bad Things Happen To Good People* (by Rabbi H.S. Kushner). The Anorexia Nervosa and Irritable Bowel Syndrome (IBS), turned paralytic, was 'managed' by diet and medications (also a form of 'Damage Control'). A 'Butterfly' morphed to a 'Turkey', Circling Mt. Doom (*Rebuilding When Your Relationship Ends* by B. Fisher), flew off it, self-transformed as an Eagle, and landed with another Eagle, as a great support, *When Bad Things Happen...* The story has been recorded, with 'Just Love' for adult children (coined in the sequel, from a prophet, to include justice with love, and matriach, to do the right thing), and with love for grandchildren, who won't know, otherwise, what they don't know (to be gifted to them at eighteen, by their grandmother, they don't know and wont meet), also in 'Just Love'.

The mentally ill doctor (first husband), was vested in the causes, more than the effects, and had pursued a CAT scan and 'Brain studies', to confirm his theory, of structural alterations, or changes in brain chemistry. As such, in the interests of further research, all proceeds of the sales of this book, shall be donated to mental health (as per the logo on the book), and where it maybe needed.

Names changed in the first book (to protect family), removed in the 'theory-based' sequel, have now been re-applied in the second edition, of ten chapters, for the events, further along the, 'Highway'.

Evidence against some of the lies, are listed in Contents as Exhibits One, Two, Three and Four.

A special edition of this book, is to be presented, with many thanks, to the Mental Health Department, Head of Mental Health, at Fremantle Hospital, Service Director of the Fiona Stanley Fremantle Hospital Group, of the South Metropolitan Health Service, Mental Health Services Doctor of Fiona Stanley Hospital, and Team Leader ATT and MHCR, of the Fremantle Hospital Mental Service.

DEDICATION

The title of the first book, and its rewritten second edition, came from the last letter, from my late ex-husband, before he walked out on the, "Reconciliation". I now pay him tribute.

"Get healthy like an Eagle, then go find another Eagle without a mental illness." (Page in Evidence as Exhibit Four). I did!

In "Regard and Honour" of my (late) parents, I thank them for doing the best they knew how. Years after their deaths, I finally understood. Thank you Dad for being my hero. Thank you Mum, for your message, "To do the right" in every card. I do the right in 'Just Love'!

Thank you, to my beloved eagle husband, for his love and support. We did the right in, "Just loving" (coined in my sequel) our children and grandchildren.

My late sibling, was my only friend, in an otherwise lonely army setting, during childhood, thank you little sister.

This edition is especially for grandchildren, who don't know what they don't know or what their grandma knows/knew. In my life, I am greatly loved, respected and honoured, by a beloved step family (their children included), thank you for your acceptance as a step mum and grandmother.

Last but not least, my only, true, best, friend, June (with permission) to stand by me for 52 years. A big thank you! Also valued, are FB Family and friends; most especially Valerie (with permission) June's sister, and a friend of my late sister.

CONTENTS

tree, indicates a second marriage for Edmund, to Maria Watkins, with a daughter born to them (presume in Ireland). Ivy was to see Edmund once, when he came to give her away, at her church wedding at St. Marks Podanur Church. Ivy had 11 children of her own, as well as two step children; including the infant son from her cousin.

Perciville Dunbar Dewar (Percy for short) was that infant son, who was not only close to his baby brother (my father), but, many times, gave Bert his heart back, when ever disappointments struck. The brothers were often seen around Podanur, with their rifles, for bird hunting, with Bert perched proudly on Percy's strong shoulders. Two of Ivy's daughters, carry the blue-eyed gene, while my father inherited the brown hair; hence the nickname, "Sandy". Bert's youngest brother Derek, also the baby of the family, was six foot tall, and the only one to inherit the height of his Irish grandfather. Bert was five foot eight when he joined the British army at eighteen.

Unique to the Dewar's, was that their father, kept the family isolated in a big house, surrounded by high walls, with locked gates. Colin was an officer of the telegraph, and claimed a descendant from gentry, and therefore superior to the people, who worked on the local railway. Although the story of a 'Lord Goth', married to an island princess, had predominated after every evening meal, all the family tree could lay acclaim to, was a three times great grandfather, named Captain William Dewar and wife Ann McLarty who were married on 25 February, 1775, in Bal-more/Baltimore Parish of Glossary, in the county of Argyll, Scotland. Being an 'officer', was reason enough, to consider his family superior and justified their isolation.

This family pride was to come to my rescue, many times over the years, as a defence to insult or rejection. Colin refused to mix with 'railway people'; anyone who worked in the British Railway, be it a guard or engine driver. Colin also raised his children self-sufficient, just as he had been, when he stuffed his punctured car tyre, full of grass, and got himself back home, from the wilderness. Perhaps it was this same pride, that compelled Bert to join the army, and overcome his homesickness, as a new recruit, crying secretly in his bed at night. This was to hold him in good stead, through a flood, and much later, through the first war, between India and Pakistan. But, he had no defences, against the beauty of Lavender Rose Brady, twelve years his junior, and the daughter of a (you guessed it) railway, engine, driver.

Lavender had not been such a beauty, in her younger days; rather more a sun-blackened "Darkie" (as the caption read on a black and white photograph), sports girl and tom-boy. Born on the 24th February, 1934 (she later tried to change into 1937 on her birth certificate), she was the first daughter of three, with three brothers (two older and one younger); a family of six, for Mavis (Stephens) and Cyril Brady. Lavender shared a special bond, with her younger, tall brother Grant, born after her, and before her youngest two sisters. My mother had relayed, many a fond memory of Mavis, as she had passed away with breast cancer, when I was three, and my younger sister Christine, just a few months old.

Mavis was 52, when she had deliberately ignored a breast lump, even after it became grossly deformed. It had already metastasised to other organs, although Cyril paid for many expensive operations, that cost Cyril his home named, "Ottoville" (sold for a pittance to Bert). Sadly, Lavender was not only unable to nurse her dying mother, but, she was limited to short visits at her sick bed, because I had chicken pox and could not be left with the 'baby ayah' for long. Mavis seemed to know and understand, Lavender's clock watching. "Go home my girl, go home to your babies", she often said to Lavender.

Mavis was a paragon of virtue, of average stature and looks, with a darker than average skin complexion. Mavis herself had been motherless at six, and raised by her eldest brother Robert Stephens (hence Lavender's third name of Roberta). Just as Mavis had

4

neglected her breast lump, so had her own mother Dr. Stephens, who neglected a cut finger, while busy doing house calls, and died from the ensuing septicaemia (blood poisoning). This is where is believed, came the aspirations, to become a doctor. Lavender was to follow in her mother's and grandmother's footsteps, of 'self-neglect'. This cycle was finally broken by me.

Lavender once recalled Mavis, eating a bowl of plain rice, long after everyone else in the household had eaten (servants included). It was this gentle, kind, softness, inherited from Mavis that was often mistaken for simplicity, naivety, ignorance, weakness or plain stupidity, causing many a family member, to use, or ill-treat Lavender, and myself (in turn). Surrounded by brothers, Lavender learned boxing, and at four foot six, could hold her own, becoming a tom-boy. When boxing didn't get Lavender out of trouble, Mavis covered up for her wild daughter's mischief.

Lavender's favourite hiding place, was the laundry basket. She would often steal mangoes from the local plantations, only to run off with the spoils, leaving her boyfriend up the mango tree, to face the plantation owner. The boy never learned his lesson, and still asked Lavender along every time. However, she was also a crack-shot, at knocking the mangoes, off the tree, so he never needed to, and refused to climb another mango tree, ever afterward. Another famous vice, Lavender was well known for, was teasing her older brother Monte, who was scared of the dark. Monte always asked Lavender, to carry the lantern, to light the way to the outside toilet (Australian 'Dunny'). Lavender waited till his pants were down, and took off, leaving Monte in total darkness. Even though she did it every time, he still asked her to go with him.

Perhaps this was how Lavender became the fastest sprinter, at her high school, and later at the Baldwin Boarding School for girls. At the boarding school, she promptly took off, with all the sports monitors and head girl, after the 'new girl'. They were unable to catch her, till she tired, and immediately demanded, she join their faction sports teams, or 'House' (as it was called) . She did, and rewarded the house she joined, with many a sports medal (the 'Darkie' photograph). So, when Lavender returned home on leave, after her first year as a nursing student, Grant did not recognise the beauty, he was sent to pick up, from the Podanur railway station. Grant was never to see that sports darkie again.

Lavender was as light skinned as her dad, a Brady except for the grey eyes (inherited by two of my cousin brothers). Lavender had fire brown eyes. Lavender's shoulder length wild hair had been tamed, cut short just like the actor Liz Taylor, she had spotted, in a fashion magazine, which had curled of it's own accord. It was to Neville, a tall Air Force pilot, her first true love, that she lost her heart. They planned to marry, after Lavender completed her nursing course. Apparently his height worked against him, when he suffered a fatal head wound, from the crushed cockpit roof of his plane, killed in action, during the Second World War. Lavender maintained, that had she not been on the rebound from Neville's death, she might never have married the serious, reserved, much older, Captain Dewar.

They met at a dance, Lavender had reluctantly attended (still heart broken). Compelled by her nursing classmate friends, Lavender went to the army dance, that Bert also happened to attend. It was to change the course of both their lives. The reserved thirty five year old was smitten, and shocked all his fellow officers, by breaking into song, on a mike, on the bandstand. Bert had had his fair share of prospects, but, the last girl had used Bert's marriage proposal, to elicit one from her long term reluctant boyfriend, whom she married. Patsy got her proposal, as soon as there was another suitor. So it was, that Bert could be forgiven, for feeling a little desperate and left on the shelf, facing permanent bachelorhood at thirty five. He was determined to marry the railwayman's daughter, against all family opposition and advice.

Lavender had earned (either deservedly or not) the unsavoury reputation of being the "Podanur Flirt". Ivy and two of Bert's oldest sisters, desperately tried to distract him, with another single,

Anglo-Indian lady, but, Heather's heart already belonged to Mally. Bert was adamant, and three short months after they met, they were secretly married in a civil ceremony. Besotted by her beauty as Bert was, he not only agreed to Lavender's request for a church wedding thereafter, but, he never let on to both families, of their civil marriage. Their engagement photograph, was actually their civil wedding photo.They were married again, at St. Marks church, by Pastor Fowler, who also happened to have been, the Principal of Baldwin Boarding school. Years later, Pastor Fowler was to correct my high school final English exam (school leaving) paper.

Lavender was already expecting me. It was at the church wedding, that Monte was to exact revenge, for all the times Lavender had run off with the lantern, leaving him in the dark, with his pants down. He was Best man and pretended to lose the wedding ring, when Pastor Fowler asked for it. Monte began to search all his pockets, with an appropriately, worried, countenance, and had his sister and brother-in-law in a big panic, before finally producing it, with a grin. Monte also told their blind (with cataracts) grandmother, that her favourite granddaughter, was marrying a black man, "dark as night". Try as she had, Lavender couldn't convince the old lady, till she saw Bert for herself, after her cataract operation.

Neither Bert nor Lavender disclosed their civil marriage, that is, until it appeared my birth was premature at seven months. Lavender already had morning sickness, which she was forced to hide, when she walked down the aisle. I was born in Madras (now Chennai) and spent my early years in Fort St. George, where I was "Christened" (named) and lumbered with three first names; one of which was removed for being miss-spelled, on all legal documents. The alternative was to prove, that the person named in the documents, was really me, over and over again.

The Christening Certificate is also a Birth Certificate. The black and white photograph, to mark the occasion, however, told a different story, according to a cousin, found on FB, five decades later. Missing was an aunt and her family; uninvited to the

7

christening, leaving an uncle and both grandmothers. Lavender had been miffed, when Susan's big sister Maureen, then just six, told Lavender off, for buying too many dresses, hand-bags and shoes, leaving uncle Bert with old, patched-up army uniforms. The six year old was no longer welcome. This rift was never healed, although Lavender saw Maureen aged sixteen, when she came for a visit with Nana Ivy.

My little sister, however, was nearly a non-entity. Lavender loved children and in her older years, played with any baby she came across, at local shopping centres. The Matron of Lavender's training hospital, forbade her to take abortive remedies, or try to get rid of her own baby. Bert had once raised doubts, over how the second pregnancy had occurred, as he had been away some months, on an army field trip. Christine was born in November, 1959, with a healthy, lusty, hungry, cry.

The difficult birth of a ten pound baby, put paid to further child-bearing for Lavender. As men were not allowed in the delivery room, and left to pace in the waiting room, Bert heard her screams from the delivery suite nearby. Bert believed sex was only meant for procreation, as such total abstinence resulted. Lavender was just twenty five. When Bert was posted to a field area, in Jammu at the foothills of the Himalayas, Lavender was sent home to 'Ottoville' with her two little girls.

Cyril Brady was overjoyed, to have his daughter and granddaughters, but, not so much his teenage daughters Ruby Rose and Jade Rose, who barely tolerated their nieces. Ruby and Jade were not a little jealous of their sister, as Nana Brady played favourites with Lavender; her pet granddaughter, with special treats of her favourite food dishes, every time the girls visited. Salt in the wound, would have been the marriage, to a well-to-do Army officer, recently promoted to a Major. The dislike was to last a lifetime. It did not seem to bother Lavender, and we saw Podanur and the Brady family, once, at the end of each year, on a months holiday. It was grandpa Cyril's cigarette butt I tried to smoke, that left me with a permanent, dislike of the habit. I was five, but, refused to go into the house, all day, for fear of anyone, smelling cigarette smoke, on my breath.

The memory of his grey eyes, twinkling above gold-rimmed glasses, as he smiled at me or teased my little sister, is much loved and cherished. It was at the Podanur Institute school, I began my education as a five year old. It was also the first time, I got away with stealing, an Indian girl's hair adornment of fresh flowers, as we both walked the short distance home. It was a grab and run, to the back gate of Ottoville, meticulously premeditated and carried out with precision. It was also possibly the time, like my mother, I learned to be a fast sprinter, stealing flowers (not mangos) and running home with the spoils, although the little girl (also my classmate) did not complain, or mention it thereafter.

However, something far more sinister, was to darken the love story of my parents, and raise even more questions than answers, about the second pregnancy, and Christine's birth. Although I was an unwitting witness to the fight, between Bert and Cyril (aged seven), I did not understand the repercussions, till many years later. It was to leave an indelible scar on their relationship, and turned out to be the perfect foliage for abuse, that was to overshadow my mostly north Indian childhood.

CHAPTER TWO

North Indian Childhood – Under Shadow

Like any couple, Bert and Lavender started out in a marriage, full of love and promise. All the earlier photographs of this period, attest to this, and their first 'love child'; their very own special "Lizzy girl". Spoiled as the first child, till Christine changed the family dynamics, as all siblings do. Cyril had warned Bert about Lavender, going out with young Naval officers, in Podanur, the reason he advised his son-in-law, to take his family to Jammu. Christine and I had been tagged along to picnics at parks, with a sailor named Clinton. Bert had defended his wife's honour, and punched Cyril (the fight I had witnessed). Grandpa Cyril's warnings, were to be proved right, not long after we arrived in Jammu. It did not take long, for Lavender to find junior officers of the six Jat (j-a-rt) Regiment, to take the Major's wife (also the wife of the second-in-command, shortened to 2-I-C), shopping in Jammu.

Jammu (now in Pakistan) is as far north, as Podanur is south, with a comfortable house, provided for the Major and his family. My mostly north Indian childhood, which had just begun, was to also reflect, my mostly north Indian Ancestry DNA (done after emigrating to Australia). 'Tamil' in the south, was replaced with 'Hindi' in the north, a much softer, sounding language with completely different letters, written below the line, arising from ancient Sanskrit roots; a form of higher Hindi. English remained the first language, after the British left. Long before we started school at 'Presentation Convent', Christine and I had mastered the Hindi language, and spoke it fluently, with other army children and orderlies. Lavender, who spoke fluent Tamil, also picked up Hindi, and spoke it well with the young officers, she went shopping with. This set the gossiping tongues a-wagging.

Bert was totally unaware, until his Quarter-master of the officers "Mess", Captain Jogindar (or Yogi, a nickname given by Lavender) Singh, suddenly stopped talking mid-sentence, when Bert walked in. After pressing the captain, Yogi spilled the beans. Apparently, Bert had been the laughing stock of the entire Regiment, for quite some time, with snickered remarks, about the Major unable to control his own wife, never mind the men in the Regiment. At five and seven, Christine and I were oblivious to the unfolding drama around us, when Bert got home, from the office that day. Lavender asked for a divorce, to marry the twenty nine year old officer, Captain Lal (l-a-rl), she had fallen in love with. Bert gave Lavender an ultimatum, she couldn't/wouldn't accept. She could have her divorce to marry her captain, provided she left without her daughters. N.B. In India, the man had full rights, to the children.

This sounded the death knoll to trust, honour, and the marriage was never the same. It also birthed the "Stronghold" of 'UN-forgiveness' for Bert, and "Negative emotions or bad things" of 'loneliness, in a loveless marriage and sense of hopelessness' for Lavender, both concepts, first identified in my sequel *Eagles On The Highway* (a reference in this book). Lavender never tried to find love again, even after both her daughters were adults. An Eagle did not repeat this mistake, when her children were adults. Lavender worked against Bert, rather than with her husband, and set out to punish Bert, instead of love him. Lavender's shopping sprees were actually, "Retail Therapy" to sublimate an inner emptiness – something an Eagle was to copy, in her unhappy marriage, and remedy with good "stewardship or money-management", in her good marriage (addressed at length in the sequel).

Oblivious to the unhappy marriage, I became 'daddy's girl' (more by accident than intent), when I joined Bert on his long, possibly therapeutic walks, after the loss of face in the Regiment, honour and a big disappointment. Christine was still too young to manage the long walks. She got tired and Bert had to carry her, for most of the first walk. So began the special bond, with a hitherto absent dad, which remains a highlight. This is where I learned about the stars, and on clear nights, still look for the Big and Little Dippers, Venus and Mars. The green countryside, with the Himalayas as a backdrop, was full of lakes and rivulets. I do regret not visiting, any of the popular mountain resorts, like Shrinagar. This is when, Bert shared his 'jungle-story', of *Assam Rifles*.

During Bert's jungle, warfare, training, leeches were a big problem. Luckily for Bert, he was a heavy smoker then, and used his lit cigarette, to burn the blood suckers off. They even managed to get under his thick, military socks. Bert also shared his survival, of a flood, when the main Brahmaputra River of Tibet, flooded it's banks, once a year, when it changed course. The water was already at chest level by midnight, when the alarm was raised. Many in the regiment drowned in their sleep. One family floated by on a mattress, past the rooftop, where Bert had clung for hours. He watched helplessly, as the entire family toppled into the raging, flood waters. As though this was not bad enough, the Chinese grabbed the wet, shivering, survivors (army personnel slept in their underwear), at the border, where the flood waters had deposited them.

Bert spun his captors a yarn, and got out, but lost his British Passport and Parker pen, gifted him by Colin Dewar, the last time he had seen his dad alive. Colin Dewar had deliberately stayed alive, through shear will-power, to see the New Year in, so that his widow would get his pension. Bert was not granted army leave, to bury his father. Bert did follow his dad's advice, to save for a rainy day, and quit smoking and drinking, "cold Turkey", to become a moderate drinker, in his late twenties. With his first savings, he was able to buy a new pair of shoes. Prior to this, Bert lived from pay to pay, as a heavy drinker and smoker. Thus the stories continued, as did the long walks.

I felt prouder still, when Bert took me to the Republic Day Parade, held on my birthday, that also happens to be "Australia Day". Bert stood on the podium, to take the 'salute' as the brigade marched past. He struck a dashing figure in khaki army greens, pressed to perfection, by his orderlies, who also shone his brass buttons, that gleamed with polish. A beret set at an angle, with the regiments insignia on the front, completed the uniform. I was even prouder, when I learned of, and saw the photograph of his, "Guard of Honour" to Prince Phillip, the Duke of Edinburgh, on the 4th February, 1959, at Dum-Dum Airport Calcutta. Bert was in full dress uniform, for this special occasion, to present the troops to the duke.

Years later, despite his heroic survival from the flood, Bert became disillusioned with the army, when he was asked to pay for his award, for saving the Indian Government, millions of Rupees, he had carefully unearthed, from the flood plane, where once had stood buildings, with army personnel. He had carefully dried out, and guarded the money, night and day. The army life did suit his daughters, and they thrived on the north Indian food, attributed to achieving a foot taller than Lavender, for both girls, and a relatively sturdy bone structure. The lentils or Dahl and large pancakes of flour, "Sooka-Roti" (dry bread) cooked on hot coals, were brought, from their canteen, by Bert's orderlies.

These orderlies were like a part of the family, and lived in a tent, beside the home. One orderly looked after Bert's uniforms, while the other fetched the food from the canteen, also for the Sahibs (Sir's) little daughters. The tent proved a great slide for Christine and me. It was one of these orderlies who interfered with me, when I was about eight, during a baby-sitting session, when Bert and Lavender, had gone out for dinner, at the officers Mess. This orderly was summarily discharged, but, I got the first beating from my father, the reason for which remains an enigma. Thus the abuse became my fault, and the dirty looks from that orderly, only served to confirm the internal dialogue of self-blame. It was to set me up for further abuse.

13

All this got pushed to the background, when war broke out, between India and Pakistan. In the confusion, Bert forgot to evacuate his own family, from the war zone. The best part was no school. Since we were the only family to remain, we were hailed as heroes, although Lavender was a reluctant one. Wearing white clothes was forbidden, and strict black-out rules applied i.e. no lights except for a candle, with the curtains drawn. A trench was dug in the backyard, with dirt steps, for swift access (in pitch darkness), during enemy, air-raids. The novelty soon wore off with sleep disturbance. I played with the stones at the bottom of the trench, as we listened, to the barely audible hum of enemy planes. The silence was only broken, by anti-aircraft guns, which lit up the sky, in a mammoth display of fireworks, tragic, when an enemy plane, got shot down in flames.

Although outside the main war zone, we were still close enough to the border, to be in danger of spies getting through. So Lavender made our guards, ask even the husbands, of the young women who stayed with us, for their papers and identification. The young wives were miffed, when their endearments were ignored, while papers were checked, but, Lavender remained resolute. Another routine established, was prayer for Bert's safety. The young Muslim and Hindu army wives often joined in the prayers, for the safety of their husbands. "War" anywhere is not nice in the least, and I can fully empathise with the Ukrainians and Russians, caught up in the current Ukraine-Russian conflict. Even though not a world war, it has affected the world, with food shortages and escalating food prices. When older, Bert told me of the catastrophe, that had unfolded on the battlefield in 1965.

The smell of burnt flesh hung in the air, dead bodies, unable to be buried, at various stages of decomposition, and body parts, lay strewn all over the battleground. In the midst of fire from rifles, tanks, bombs and hand grenades, many a private turned and ran from their post – the officer in charge included. It had taken a lot of fast talking, by Bert, to woo these deserters back. If Bert shot every deserter, he wouldn't have had any men left, to lead into battle. Bert did not shame his superior either. He just told the men, the Commander, Colonel Jug was already wounded in battle, and a hero. Thereafter, as the 2-I-C, he not only took command, but, made a huge noise, as he led the men, so they could hear he was with them. Jug got all the credit, but, Bert remains my hero. The bond forged on the long walks, was to hold me in good stead, in the rejections ahead.

Princess Joti of Kashmir, had been a classmate in grade three, taught by Lavender. The princess was also tutored, at her palace by Lavender. I never did learn what became of this princess after the war. Not long afterwards, Bert was posted to an Army Recruitment Centre, in Secunderabad, a twin city of Hyderabad (where international cricket matches are played). Bert was given a huge British style built home for his family, in Trimulgherry, on the outskirts of Secunderabad. I was nine and because of home schooling by Lavender, considered to be advanced for my age, and promoted to a grade higher at the St. Ann's convent. Christine was put in her regular class. St. Ann's was conveniently located close to Bert's recruiting office. Telegu was as foreign a language, as the much warmer climate and red earth tones and was never learned.

Hindi was still the main second language, which got the family by in the marketplace, and available in school. Schools were open for half day (till one p.m.) on Saturdays, Sunday was the only day off for homework. There was one difficult teacher (Miss Couper in fifth grade was the meanest) and I fought my sister's battles. All that running practice in Podanur now paid off. I hit the classmates, that dared to bully Christine (at recess), and took off like the wind. If they had big sisters, I ran faster. I was my mother's daughter after all.

Bert decided to put us in boarding school, at the age of eleven and nine. The army school of Laurence in Lovedale, was in the Nilgiri Hills. Built by the British, with a high reputation, it was not far from Podanur. I hated the regimented lifestyle, although Christine thrived on it, and the independence. It was at this school, I first heard of my look-alike cousin Susan, I was to meet, along with her dad Dennis, in Podanur, not long afterward. As mentioned I found her again, on FB, thanks to another cousin Sandra, who passed away, two short years after re-connecting with her. Susan and I share another bond, of a common hatred for this school. Mrs Gupta, the headmistress of our dormitory, was cruel to Christine, and forced her to eat the foods, she could not tolerate, such as tomatoes and eggplant (that have seeds). Christine promptly vomited all over the dining table, and was sent to bed without supper.

The only highlight, in the three month boarding school experience, was the first taste of having a boyfriend; sixteen year old Nicholas Horsebro, a bugle-playing, blonde, curly haired, upper-school boy, with the deepest of dimples. Although we never spoke, he sent sweets from 'Nic', amidst many blushes, for being teased about, 'liking' each other. This was not enough to quell the rising homesickness. The first opportunity to go home, came at the first visit to the school, by Bert and Lavender. It met with failure, as I clung to my mothers legs, begging to go home, Mrs Gupta ordered my parents off the school grounds, leaving me to her repercussions. She boldly took the chocolate cake, I won in a raffle, not long afterward.

Mrs Gupta also stole our tuck boxes and parcels from home. Letters, to and from home, were edited. I finally got the chance, to tell Lavender the truth, when she came on a solo visit, a month later. Bert could not bear the sight of his pining wife, and gave in to her request to visit, knowing full well she would bring her girls home. He was not surprised, to see the three of us disembark from the train, when he came to pick Lavender up. Sadly, the bitterness between Bert and Lavender, took a turn for the worse, with frequent, angry fights, invariably over money and overspending. This is when, Christine and I got roped into the "Game"; a cruel conspiracy, of sneaking money out of Bert's trunk, saying, "What dad didn't know, couldn't hurt him". She cleverly found the key, to unlock the trunk, and stole the notes from the middle of the pile, as Bert kept the serial numbers, of the first and last notes. Lavender taught her girls to steal.

The affair with a neighbour's husband, however, cost us the friendship, with the Cur family. There was no more playing "Cowboys and Indians" with Patrick, Michael and Judy. No more invites to birthday parties either, or invites to the Cur kids to our big birthday parties, put on by Lavender. Also lost, was the special new game of 'dark room hide and find'. When goats got into the compound, through open gates, Christine and I, missed their help, in chasing them out. Cricket with the boys had also been fun, especially as a top runs scorer, even though a girl. They made the mistake, of throwing the ball gently, but, soon realised it, and tried to get me out. All three children were sent off to Keti (kay-tee), a civilian, sister, boarding school of Laurence, never to be seen again. Years later, there was brief contact with Patrick on FB, but, it fell away to silence.

In grade nine, there was a choice between two streams of study: arts or science. I chose science, as I already knew I wanted to be a doctor. This notion was first conceived, after a minor operation to remove a splinter, from my right pointer finger, at the army hospital nearby. After the operation, a new game of hospitals emerged, with dolls as the patients, who were injected with water coloured by crepe paper, from Christmas decorations. The green one tasted the worst of course. The dolls were soon covered with holes from their injections, much as was pumped into my thirteen year old, skinny, arms (as teenagers didn't have injections anywhere else), for ten days, to quell the infection in my finger, and avoid the aforementioned surgery. Instead of abating, after two courses of antibiotics, the infection spread up the arm. So it was, that my very first general anaesthetic, inspired medicine, as well as perhaps, also my late, great, grandmother Dr. Stephens.

The science stream was far more difficult, than its arts counterpart, and my double promotion in grade five, began to bite. It was specifically a struggle, with maths and English comprehension. Enter, *The Famous Five* and *The Secret Seven* series, by Enid Blyton which (now grace the bookshelves of my step-grandsons), improved comprehension and vocabulary; the beginnings of my writing as an author. It birthed the new love of reading and writing (that still remains), and was a solace, escape and sublimation, of my social life. My gift of 'Writing' was thus born. All school friends lived an hours drive away, even my new best friend Veena Marwah. Half-day school on Saturday's and church all Sunday, left no time for sleepovers. Bike riding around Trimulgherry, till the street lights were lit, was the only outlet, other than the open air cinema, at the army club every Thursday, or Hindi movie every Monday, i.e. if the weather held.

It was Maths homework, that was to bring back a crushing memory, especially when Lavender said and did nothing, again, as I was to do, when the father of my children, beat them (now recognised as abuse, not discipline). The beatings solidified the bad self-belief, as well as stupid, with acceptance that Bert merely wanted better for me. He had missed the first six years of school and teachers had called him a dummy. As adults, Colin had compared Bert with his university educated sister; a sibling rivalry to be repeated, to some extent, with his own daughters. Exactly what *Family Of Origin* (course done) is made of.

Bert had also struggled with study, to become an officer. Each time Bert began calmly enough, but, the blows soon fell painfully, across the shoulder blades or head. "Two twos are six?" he demanded, as he yanked my ear, already red, swollen and painful, from the head blows, by strong, army-trained, muscled, arms. On one occasion, I begged for mercy, as I wet my pants, adding embarrassment to the list. Every time, Bert would apologise, with money, only to re-offend.

The beatings and blood blisters, did not stop, because Bert had seen the error of his ways. They stopped, because six months into the school term, the maths problems became too difficult, and

I was able to show him, how it was done. By this time, I had endured beatings, on an almost daily basis. This drove an Eagle, to become a high achiever at university level, with a research unit employed, to formulate the concepts and theories, proposed in the sequel, and applied to this continuing story. However, another evil in the form of "improper touching" began with the Hindi tutor, Bert found in his subordinate officer. It was scheduled every morning, for an hour before school, to help with "Sanskrit", now a part of the science stream. It looked and sounded like Hindi, but, could have come from an Egyptian tomb of a Pharaoh, for all the sense it made.

I did not want yet another beating, so kept silent, till the tuition stopped abruptly, for as yet an unknown reason. Looking back, I think this had a lot to do, with Bert not getting a promotion, or extension of service. I did not speak up again, when a trusted family friend, and church elder, groomed and won his paedophilia-prize, by stealing a first kiss. Sixty year old Mr. Vivekanundar, was clever, but, thankfully, I was able to avoid his advances, when realisation dawned, on what he intended, after learning the facts of life, from his eldest, soon-to-be-wed, daughter. The whole family, were invited to the wedding, as close friends, but, neither Bert nor Lavender suspected a thing. I was too ashamed, to share this dirty secret, with my Temple-going, Sikh, best friend Veena, or any of my other deeply, religious, Hindu, girlfriends. I didn't confide in Lavender either, even though she had been the only one, to hear my plea, to take me out of boarding school.

It was about this time, that Bert hoped to make full Colonel, and applied for a five year army extension. Neither was granted, due to an indiscretion by Bert, reported by his junior officer (presume the same one who abused me, or coveted Bert's position, after his retirement). Thus disappointed, Bert permitted Lavender to apply to Canada and Australia, for emigration. Australia replied, thanks to Jade Brady's sponsor (the first of the Brady family to emigrate with her ex-navy husband). In hindsight, I owe this aunty, a debt of gratitude, for sponsoring and supporting my family, as new migrants.

Jade was to sponsor all her siblings. Grant settled in Melbourne, in Victoria; the Eastern States of Australia. Eldest brother Ray, Monte and Ruby came to Perth, Western Australia. So, although we had approval, we became the last, as Bert and Lavender, decided to wait the two years required, for me to finish high school (school leaving). Not unlike the family had done every December, for a month's holiday, since arriving in Secunderabad, the blue (a favourite colour of Bert's and mine) Ambassador car, was packed for the last and final three-day drive, via Bangalore, back to Podanur, and Ottoville, for the last two years in India. This was a form of a final exodus, for the Brady Clan, and most of the Dewar Clan. It was also part of a mass exodus of Anglo-Indians, from India to England, Canada, the U.S.A and of course Australia.

CHAPTER THREE

The Final Exodus

Podanur to the the Dewar girls, only meant parties, sports carnivals, and dances over the festive season. It only felt strange, when the month passed, and there was no return to Secunderabad. Also different, was no Brady family, as uncle Grant and his family, were already in Melbourne and Grandpa Cyril had passed away. I recall with fondness the last time we saw grandpa, when he had remarked how tall I was, even at eleven (cousin Susan is also tall). Grandpa was to come, for a holiday to Secunderabad, before he left with uncle Ray, for Australia. Bert had unilaterally cancelled this trip, leaving Lavender devastated. Cyril died in hospital, waiting for Lavender. Lavender and her girls did attend the funeral. Ray's three children, played cruel games, by running and hiding, from Christine and me. They remain estranged.

Ruby Brady stayed briefly, till she caught her flight out to Perth, with her son and husband. All the Brady clan, except Jade, borrowed their air fares, as a mutual benefit to Bert, to take money out of India, where it was repaid in dollars. This bypassed the cash restrictions, on immigrant families, even though Bert had to wait a year or two. Lavender was in her element, and well known for her fashion and dress sense, while we were referred to as, 'Lavender's daughters'. Our family again attended St. Marks church, where my parents had been married in 1956, by Mr Fowler, who was still the pastor. Lavender, his favourite ex-student, became the Sunday school teacher.

Without cousins, all the children in Sunday School, became our friends very quickly, as letters to Veena, finally died a natural death, a few months later. Decades later, a dream placed Veena in the outback of Australia. Carol singing was the big event of the season, beginning with choir practice. Annabelle, Geraldine, and their nineteen year old, big brother Ray Lemearl (in-laws of uncle Grant), invited the Dewar girls, to go carol singing, around Podanur. Ray kissed my neck, but, when a girl friend emerged, he was dumped, in public, on the dance floor. That's all a thirteen year old, could think to do at the time. The gossip had it, that his girlfriend had had an abortion, but, as this was never confirmed, it did not change the stance made, at the ball.

At the New-Year's Ball, the new Dewar girls were most popular, with all the Anglo-Indian boys. I danced with three or four at a time. The boyfriend in Secunderabad, had been of the briefest of encounters, meeting once, at the army club and long-distance, phone chats, from a neighbours phone. There's little doubt, Vinod would've gone back, to my ex-friend Sumedha Sahani, as soon as I left. The neighbour's prophecy, about a future husband bears mention: "Look at the heart, not looks of the man you will marry. You will be very pretty, a beautiful woman. If you choose a good-hearted man, you will be happy. Choose good looks and you will be miserable". The Eagle's story bears out this prophecy, with one of each. Reading Barbara Cartland love novels, set the scene, for a good looking, knight, in shining armour.

Then I saw the choir boy, who did not seem able to take his eyes off me, all through the service. Harold Hawk was a skinny, tall boy of fourteen, with light brown hair and a fair complexion. He stood out in his red and white St. Marks choir boy outfit. He had just returned from Keti. Harold was to become the third boyfriend, after Nicholas and Vinod. For a thirteen year old, it was a case of 'out of sight, out of mind', after Harold kissed me goodbye (my first kiss from a boy), at the back gate of Ottoville, before he left to return to Keti. When Harold returned from Keti, the Hawk's and Dewar's played a game called 'Seven Tiles'. A stack of seven flat stones, had to be hit apart by a tennis ball, which started the game for two teams; one to rebuild, and the other to prevent it being rebuilt, by hitting "out" just one team member, with the tennis ball, passed between team mates. It was Harold's team versus Liz's Team, but both belonged to the "Thunder Birds Club". The leaders were T1 and T2.

Also in Keti, were June (my best friend) and her younger sister Valerie, both similar in age, became friends with Christine and me. I first met June at St. Marks, where her family attended. Her younger brother and sisters also attended Sunday School. June is a gentle, quietly spoken, home-body, the direct opposite of a vivacious, talkative, effervescent, thirteen year old, I had been at the time. When ever Harold was home, he would call for me, on the way to church or Sunday school. Lavender put on a church play for St. Marks that first Christmas, back in Podanur and the next. It is unknown who took over from Lavender, after we left India.

All the Sunday School children mucked, around (as children do), during rehearsals, and even made fun of a carol, singing, "While shepherds washed their socks at night, all seated around the tub, a cake of soap came tumbling down, and they began to scrub", instead of "While shepherds watched their flocks by night, all seated on the ground, an angel of the Lord came down, and glory shone around". But we came through for Lavender on the day. Harold's humble, box, camera, took the only (black and white) photographs, that survived the burning of photographs, years later. There was history between a Hawk and a Dewar, in that Harold's dad nearly married, my aunty. We determined to break the curse, or bad karma of the past.

St. Francis convent, Coimbatore, was to be the last convent, attended for both Dewar girls. As a new girl, in her final two years, of high school, and fifteen not sixteen, academia and academic associates were chosen, as well established click groups, were difficult to get into, in the last two years of school.

Candy who attended St. Marks, was in my class, but, already had a long term best friend named Barbara. I ate lunch alone. I knew I had to finish well, to get into medicine, in Australia and put all energy into study. My electives of Geometry, Trigonometry and Algebra (akin to Maths II), seemed easier (possibly because there was a Pre-University-Course or PUC year, before college, which did in effect, make my high school pass equal to a 'Fourth Year' and not school leaving as supposed). Had I known, I would have stayed for it too. Someone once told me, that you can't put an old head on young shoulders. A fourth year was to serve my purposes.

The grades got better and I ended third in my class out of over fifty students. Winning the May Queen Ball, was yet another achievement. But the inner voice taunted, 'pretty dumb', it was Bert's, and a pretty dumb, "Butterfly" (on the cover) was born, but, ended a strong, confident Eagle, at peace with herself. Its a case of Live-In-Peace, or LIP rather than RIP. Bert also told me, that I was ever only good enough to be a Teacher (no offence intended to all Teachers) and smart, ugly, Christine was the doctor. At the time, Harold had been the lone voice, who respected me as a beautiful and smart woman. Then I missed three months of high school in my final year, due to jaundice, a side effect of bowel adhesions (I hazard a guess as a nurse), after the removal of my Appendix .

Christine had no such side effect after her Appendectomy. The servant or ayah, gave me a herb to drink, at sunrise, and put me on a diet of oranges, termed "sweet limes" in India, as mandarins are Indian 'oranges'. I've hated oranges ever since. Bert was proved wrong, when I passed with a first class, with distinctions in Maths and surprise of surprises, Hindi and a 'B' in English (thank you Mr. Fowler). My Hindi tuition Master, took all credit, although I had by-hearted all twenty essays, and spat out five for the exam. So much for that dumb label from Bert. My two week study plan and silent prayer, had paid off.

After the final exams, I finally allowed excitement back, as I looked forward to going to the land of promise. I could not have known or guessed, that the last black and white Photograph, Harold took of my family of four, with his box camera, would come to represent, the last time the family would be together. It was not going to Australia or Australia itself, that fractured the family, but, the adaptations and adjustments that resulted, from the uprooting, one country to another. Long gone was the fancy dress ball, where an Anglo-Indian, painted himself, as a gold statue, head to toe, startling Lavender, as he stood still in the ballroom. As soon as he won the prize, he had hot-footed it home, for a turps wash.

Also gone was old Mrs Golding, who had to watch out for prankster, young, Anglo-Indian, boys, putting her pot plants, at the local toilet block. Widowed early and with six young children to feed, she was well known for her big, 'Doggie Bags' (more a sack than a bag), at parties, to feed her brood. Although everyone laughed at her, June and I had been respectful to Mrs Golding, feeling sorry for her. She became so stingy, she forgot how to give, even to her own children. She ended up alone, abandoned and forgotten, and all her precious, gold, jewellery, stolen. All her children are in Australia. Her son married my aunt.

Most poignant of all, was the last day in Podanur. There were many last-timers, that December of 1972. Harold came over to Ottoville to say "farewell", not goodbye. He gave me a cheap, dress ring, as a token of our engagement, till he could come and give me a real one, when his family emigrated to Melbourne. I stayed in Harold's arms, kissing and cuddling, till it was time to leave for the Podanur, train station. A final goodbye was to be repeated once, thirty years later, and then, never to meet again. The station was full of memories of Cyril.

Lavender must have pictured him as a guard again, waving his flags at the engine driver; old Mr. Timmins with his Australian jokes of "frill cakes" for hoppers. They once held up the train, for

Lavender to be on time for Stane's School. It was these students, who had teased convent girls, mercilessly, for the long, daggy, bloomers and sports-skirts; worn down to our knees, the nuns had insisted on. Bert struck a good figure, for a retired army officer of fifty, while Lavender at thirty eight was still beautiful, looking years younger (changing her DOB would've been justified). With her departure, had also left the 'Lady of Fashion' of Podanur. She once mixed pale blue with purple for a Christmas dress, that was copied immediately. As the train pulled out, tears ran down my cheeks, and Harold's hand slipped from mine. "Write to me", my first true love shouted, as he yelled the postcode, for Podanur. We flew out from Madras or Chennai after an overnight stay in Singapore. The last Brady had left town.

CHAPTER FOUR

Coming To Australia

We landed at midnight, at Perth International Airport, on Christmas day, 1972, in our best, tailor-made, pant-suits in purple, orange and blue, alongside a smartly suited Bert. Carrying our matching handbags, with matching scarves, we were all directed to the 'New immigrants desk' and lots of paper work. Jade and Monte Brady, met us outside the customs office, and drove us, for what seemed an interminable period of time, which we later realised, was the Freeway, to a Fremantle block of flats, situated in front of the Anzac Monument, facing the sea port and off the main High Road. Jade was in a ground floor flat, and rented a two bedroom flat, on behalf of Bert, on the first floor. Christmas cake was served, as we sat glued to the black and white television (T.V.), even the advertisements were exciting.

Bert and Lavender, eventually had to tear their daughters, away from the T.V. The flat felt cramped, after Ottoville, with it's large compound. The Anzac Monument, behind our flat, served as a sign post, as we got our bearings, of the lay out. Bert and Lavender got to do their own shopping at the supermarket, very different to servants going to market each day. The Christmas service in the Fremantle church, left us cold and unwelcome, much as the Easter one did the following April. Letters from Harold had brought little comfort. At fifteen, I was cheap labour and was first to get a job, at a leather good store called, "Dreske' – Somorf". The job entailed gluing hems and seams, to be sewn by the seamstress. My slow English drawl, with different annunciations, was misinterpreted by the owner, Mrs Somorf, for being 'slow', stupid and a tad, ignorant and she talked down to me. My first experience of a "Hire-Purchase-Scheme" was to buy a vacuum cleaner and stereo for Lavender, to play her favourite, Jim Reeves records.

While I withdrew into a cloak of proud, silence, thirteen year old Christine simply answered, "Planet earth" to the question of her 'country of origin'. Myers in Fremantle, laid the foundation for an inferiority complex, after being served absolutely last, having waited at the counter, for over twenty minutes. It was good to give up the job, to return to school, when it was first learned, the High School Diploma, was only a 'Fourth year' equivalent. Neither Ray Brady, a teacher at John Curtin High School, nor Jade, had bothered to advise Lavender, although Jade could be forgiven as a new mum. Disappointed, but, not phased, I was enrolled in fifth year, and Christine in second year. I found the curriculum, at John Curtin too confusing, as some subjects were known, while others drew a blank. A bad situation worse, was the frustration, of not being understood or understanding any teachers, with my speech punctuated by many a "Pardon?"

All this paled in comparison, to what Christine was put through, on her first day at John Curtin High school. Much darker in complexion (possibly the reason Bert called her ugly), her classmates pushed her around in a circle of girls, in the locker room, as they chanted racial slurs at her, such as "Wog". I only learned of this horror, when Christine told me, years later. Ray's children, our cousins, were in school, but, ignored us as did our uncle. Remarkably, there was one, solitary exception, Anne, a tall, blonde, student who extended warmth and friendship, to both Dewar sisters, when every one else shunned them. Incidentally, Ann was to become my sister-in-law, five years later, also a bridesmaid at my wedding.

After Jade complained to her sister, about the rude disrespect of both nieces, we never went to her flat again. In hindsight, after having my own children, I could understand what it would've been like, to have two teenage nieces around, a first time mum with a baby, just a few months old. I took Jade's rejection hard, as she was all the family, we had had close by (and in the light of uncle Ray's indifference). Also gone was our stay-at-home mum. Lavender returned to nursing, or tried to. She had to do a three month, nursing orientation course, which stretched to a year. She struggled with the course, because she had contrived her certificates, from people she knew, rather than work as a nurse. She hadn't worked a day, since her training in Madras/Chennai, and was rusty and out-of-date. Although light skinned like me, with a name like Dewar, she had to explain Anglo-Indian, many times over, in her nursing career (as I was also soon to do).

Bert applied for a job as a store man. Each time he attended the interview, he was knocked back. They liked the name, but, not the brown man that turned up, for the interview. An officer, once in the British army, and escorted a prince on parade, ended up as a factory hand, in a mattress making factory, called 'Dunlop'. Bert learned to laugh off, the many derogatory terms applied to him, by rough, factory hands, namely "Wog" and "black bastard". Bert gave as good as he got, for nearly twenty years, even though it hurt his pride, thumbs and finger tips, often split and bleeding, covered in band-aids. He never complained, as the head of the family and 'Bread-winner', and I respected him anew. Ultimately, his loyalty made him a valued and respected worker, so much so, the CEO offered him an extension, after retirement (age of sixty-five). Bert refused the factory's offer to delay retirement. The Dewar pride had served him well. Bert bought his first car; a two-door, orange, Holden Torana.

I gave up study at John Curtin, after a few months, pretended to go to school, only to hide at the monument, till school gave out. I returned to the flat, when Bert got home from the factory. When the winter rains became unbearable, I was compelled to confess. A worse fate awaited, in the form of Secretary College at Fremantle TAIFE. By the time Bert enrolled me, I had missed three months of shorthand and typing, and was expected to catch up, in my own time. From that day to this, I hate both, and only do it two fingered, for phones and laptops, as an absolute necessity. After a half-hearted attempt to catch up, I gave up again, and applied for a full time job, in a Coles supermarket, in Claremont. Parents were told it was part-time. The ever growing internal dialogue now included, bad, stupid, dumb, inferior, brown, migrant. The land of milk and honey had soured and turned very bitter.

Another chapter in abuse, came to a close. The circumstances are somewhat vague, but, I recall Christine and I were bickering, as sisters do. Bert's solution, was the infamous hit, across the shoulder blades, delivered with stinging accuracy. It hurt like hell, but, I refused to cry or cower, and looked him straight in the eyes, with compressed lips, that trembled slightly. I refused to give Bert the satisfaction and my dad never hit me again. I was sixteen, and Bert knew he had crossed a line. Six months later, sometime after a lonely, first Easter, I met my novel, *white knight in shining armour*. Lavender's love books, were about to get me in a whole mess of trouble. Also, I could not bring myself to share my shameful failures, in letters to Harold. He was still in Podanur, and I needed his respect.

Dale Meade came into our lives, via a mutual friend of both families, an Anglo-Indian named Michael Jaxon. Mr. Jaxon had migrated a few years earlier, and was famous for his wedding under a 'Tamarind tree'. It had been Dale, who had showed the most interest, in the new migrants from India. Aged nineteen, Dale was a second year medical student, at the University of W.A. (UWA). He was tall, dark and handsome, with double-lashed hazel eyes, as be-fitted a knight. It was later established, that he descended from the original Fremantle Meade brothers. This claim is supported by a history book, held at the main Fremantle Library. Dale invited the Dewar family, to the Fremantle Church of Christ.

I was smitten, and dear sweet, loving, loyal, letter-writing Harold was forgotten, when Dale called to pick me up for church. It was easily better than the cold church in the Fremantle square. Dale kept the confidence, of my full time supermarket job for years, till I was ready to disclose it. He became my only friend, and had lunch with me at a park, near my supermarket, which was not far from UWA on the Stirling Highway. On one occasion, Dale bought a tub of yoghurt, he could ill afford, on his student allowance, just so he could speak with me at the checkout. He promptly sat on it, in his old bomb (car) when about to drive back to his university.

The Dewar sisters finally found acceptance and welcome in this church. At about this time, when I showed an interest in Dale's guitar, he gave me lessons. As Dale couldn't hold a tune, and I played better than Dale (having more time than a medical student), Dale generously presented me with his guitar, which touched my heart. Dale's divorce' mum Mrs Iris Meade and my family, began to alternate lunch. Dale's older sister Gale, was a nurse in Tasmania, having left home at sixteen. Younger brother Maxwell (Max) at seventeen, had dropped out of high school and worked at the Commonwealth Bank, and I had already met little sister Anne. They lived in a duplex nearby.

Dale's father Lewis, had the family home, in Hilton, after the divorce. Dale was seventeen and had obviously developed a strong bond with his mother. I believed this to be a good omen, as if he treated his mother well, it followed, he would treat his wife well too. It was always Dale who did the dishes at home. He laid the table, helped with the meal, did the family laundry, and was a general handy-man around the house. Old, retired mechanic, Mr. Hubbard, a neighbour, helped the young medical student, with repairs on his old Austin Lancer. So, as his friend, I got to help with his car, chores, and part time jobs, rolling and delivering newspapers and gardening. Iris worked as a secretary, to the Deputy head of Fremantle Hospital. She was a 'shorthand' expert. Most important of all, Dale paid board.

My introduction to the Australian cuisine, came from Iris. Salads, I first called "cow-food", replaced the Anglo-Indian curries, Irish, Dumpling and brown stews. The chicken curry didn't taste the same; a huge difference between free-range chickens, and thawed out ones, much like free-range eggs and caged, eggs. Ice-cream was no 'biggie'. We always had Lavender's home-made ice-cream, as we could afford a fridge. Bert had sacked the 'Dhobi', and bought a washing machine, to train the women of the house, to do their own laundry. Bert missed his first car (sold before emigrating), but, we missed the four doors more. I promised myself a four-door, first car. Bert bought the cheapest bedroom furniture, with regret for selling, solid centuries old Rosewood furniture, instead of bringing it. Again, left ill-advised by Jade, Monte or Ray, although both brothers were quick enough, to ask to borrow their airfares.

My first friend was thirteen year old, Julie (nicknamed 'Jewels') Andrews, who had set her heart on, twenty year old Elton John, in the group. I took the younger girl to heart, as a precious jewel and little sister. As I became more involved with Dale, Harold receded in my affections and thoughts. Perhaps I was my grandfather Colin Dewar's granddaughter after all, when I began to entertain thoughts of marriage, to a white, doctor, instead of an Anglo-Indian, still in high school. A doctor would be far more capable, of keeping me, and the family we would have, to the standards, to which I had become accustomed. Looking into becoming a nurse, completed the fantasy, of a nurse-doctor romance, often read about, in those damn Barbara Cartland novels! Dale became the tall, white, knight, in shining armour, of the "novel love story" in my head.

Then I sent Harold that horrid, "Dear John" letter, to break up with him, so I could pursue Dale. In the break-up letter, I said I was going out with Dale (a lie). Harold wrote back, to say he still loved me, if I loved him and wouldn't move on, with another girl in Keti. I did reply with a page full of, "I love you", and entrusted it to Christine, to mail on my behalf. Unknown for seven years, till Christine told me, was that she never posted that letter. A Dewar to the core, she decided, a doctor was better than a trainee train-driver, now in Melbourne. Harold receded further in thought, when I had just been accepted for nursing, by Royal Perth Hospital (R.P.H); one of three training hospitals. My St. Francis High school certificate, was declared equivalent to a 'Fourth Year' and accepted for the diploma. Nursing seemed to be the natural alternative to medicine. I went directly from check-out-chic, to student nurse, without resigning from the supermarket. Again, Dale was the only one who knew.

If I couldn't be a doctor, I would marry one. When I hadn't heard from Harold, in a month; the customary time it took a letter to reach S. India, I declared my love for Dale. Dale's reply was to come back to mock me, years later. He said he was not sure, because he was on an amber/orange light; as in "Traffic Lights". Dale later shared, that his mother had told him, that there were plenty of fish in the sea, and he didn't have to be so serious about a girl, he was just dating. However, Dale said he never wanted to lead any girl "Up the garden path". Our first, official, date, was the second-year medical ball. I asked Lavender for money for our date, but, Lavender smiled as she assured me, that the boy paid. Then I went to sit in the back seat, not wanting to be a 'fresh' sixteen year old, but, there was a hole in the floor. Musically tone deaf, with two left feet, Dale was instructed with a "One, Two, Three", for the very first dance. Dale was a fast learner, but, needed the count, whenever we danced, thereafter.

The second date, was a movie called *Godspell*. Resplendent in a long dress, I had sewn from a pattern, and Dale in his best date attire, the Austin Lancer, we named *Buttons* broke down. Dale already had a reputation, for being late to lectures, often with grease-blackened hands, after fixing his car, on the side of the Highway. As Dale's face flushed red with embarrassment, I pushed and he restarted the car. Six months later, Dale bought tickets to the play entitled *The Golden Gondoliers*.

This is when the "accidental hand holding", happened. It was during intermission, and as Dale got up to get us an ice-cream cone, I reached out to grab his jacket, (as he hadn't heard over the din), to wait for me. The hand slipped, and Dale kept hold of it, without a word. Later, I had insisted on an explanation, that I was neither fresh nor forward. So began the hand-holding, and a "Novel, imitation, love story", at the same time I began nursing. I was as an 'Australian Citizen', (now forty eight years ago), and the proud owner of a friendship ring.

CHAPTER FIVE

Nursing Chose Me
and
A Novel 'Imitation' Love Story

Nursing 'chose' me, because instead of medicine, I was only academically, equipped to do nursing. There were three classes a year. Mine was the first in January, 1974 (1/74), five days before my seventeenth birthday, with special permission, as all ninety students, were the stipulated age of seventeen and a half, or older. It was in the days, when trained nurses were addressed as 'Sister'. Sister Bloom (we didn't dare use her first name), with her long, white veil, pinned neatly and precisely atop her silver hair, earned me my nickname of *Andy Cap*, by instructing me to wear my student-nurse hat forward, towards my forehead, while the rest of the nurses, wore it on their crowns. Our first lesson, was to make a proper hospital bed. All beds had to line up perfectly with the pillow slips pointing in the correct direction. I still make my bed with hospital corners 'hospital style'.

Student nurses got their 'baptism' into the nursing diploma, in the "Pan Room". My first pan room was on ward two, in the old section of R.P.H, on the second floor. It was a medical ward, mainly for older patients, with medical conditions, such as Strokes, heart attacks, Emphysema etc. It was on ward two, that I was to have my first experience, of a dying patient (with emphysema). I watched aghast, as Mr. Smith began to gurgle, with eyes bulging, as he gasped for air. He reached out to me, but, I turned and ran to the office, to report it to the charge nurse. Mr. Smith was in one of three critically ill patient beds, next to the office, with a glass window for observing these patients. The charge nurse had seen Mr. Smith. She drew the curtains around Mr. Smith, as he turned a dusky grey. I have often wished, I was brave enough, to hold his outstretched hand, as he died.

Mr. Smith had been a heavy smoker, and paid a terrible price. I was suddenly glad I hadn't taken up the habit, and silently thanked grandpa Cyril, for that cigarette butt. Christine started at thirteen, possibly for social acceptance, and remained a heavy smoker, till her death. Dale was a non-smoker too, unlike his father, brother and younger sister. My second ward was ward three, on the third floor, of the old block, with a specialised unit called a "Life Island", for patients with Leukaemia. At just sixteen, her long nails were painted a brilliant red, in direct contrast to her pallor, fragile frame and wasting body. Cindy was being 'Reverse-barrier' nursed, in this Island. Everything in the unit had to be sterilised. Her visitors had to cap, gown, glove and mask up. Cindy had to be protected from all infections, as even a cold, could kill her. Every shift I worked, I asked if she was still there, till one morning she wasn't. Just a year younger, she showed me how to die with dignity and courage.

I did not want to associate, with other Asian student nurses, in our class and went after the white students, with an over-the-top, bubbly, people-pleasing, happy persona, directly opposite to the one used, as a defence at Dreske'-Somorf. I netted Blondy, Sherry and Maria, but, all came as 'package deals'. Blondy had Elizabeth or 'Lizzy' from primary school days, also in our class. So I was now 'Liz' to distinguish one Elizabeth from another. Sherry came with Fergie, and Maria had Sarah. Blondy and Jewels were to last only nineteen years, but, not the distance. The reason is purported to be connected, to believing lies of a white doctor, which discredited a brown nurse.

It is also believed to be, connected to liars who played 'Blaming Games' (for a suicide included), due to mental illness (from *The Road Less Travelled* by psychiatrist Dr. M. S. Peck a reference in the sequel and in this edition). Other casualties, came to include a Curtin university lecturer in the 'Nursing faculty' (now Population Health) and a co-university student from Africa. It had had the added benefit of "Isolation and control". As discussed in my sequel, if friendships are not two-way, then they go 'No-way'! My only friends remain June (my best friend), who emigrated to New Zealand (N.Z) and her sister Valerie, who emigrated to Canada.

Towards the end of first year (of three), night duty reared its ugly head. I had only just gotten used to sleep deprivation, between a late and early shifts. A morning shift began at 7a.m and ended at 3.30p.m. The afternoon started at 2.30p.m, and ended at 11p.m. (with a half hour for hand-over). All first year students, had the unenviable task, of emptying drainage bags, before going off-duty. This made for a much later knock-off time, particularly, if it became hectic as it often did, sometimes as late as 11.30p.m. At first I had to catch a bus from Fremantle, in front of the Target store, at 5a.m; an hour and a half away from R.P.H. It was much easier, when Bert purchased a three bedroom unit in South Perth. Bert gave me rides, to and from R.P.H, but it was still a good half hour drive home. I was lucky if I got six hours sleep. On a positive note, it was good for continuity of patient care, as the same patients (now 'clients') were re-allocated the next morning.

Night duty began at 9.30p.m, and went through to 7.30a.m. It was the longest nursing shift. The first challenge, was keeping awake for the very first night, after just an afternoon nap or no nap at all. Bewitching hour was around 2a.m. The only way to stop falling asleep in the office, was to do a round of the patients and have a strong coffee. As a stimulant, this added to the trouble of sleeping the next day, with noisy neighbours, and day-light filtering through closed drapes. This changed for the worse, when I got my drivers licence at eighteen, and I drove myself home, fighting sleep all the way. Some nurses have accidents, falling asleep at the wheel, while driving home, after night duty.

The other advantage, was weight loss. As the teenage 'puppy fat' dropped off, so had the friendship ring, lost after six months. Christine moved to the South Perth High school, and found a friend in Vonnie. When the South Perth youth group, rejected Christine, as a girlfriend and marriage prospect, she turned to drugs and parties. I was far too busy, with nursing and Dale, to notice the yawning gap developing, since I left John Curtin. Thankfully, she had Vonnie, who knew what she was into, that Lavender unwittingly funded. Vonnie became like a third sister, and was one of my bridesmaids. Sadly, Vonnie had passed away, before Christine's first marriage.

My first car was a new, lemon, *four-door* Datsun 120Y. I had had plenty of practice, with a very patient Bert, to and from all nursing shifts. My first driving lesson began on the Canning Highway, with a very brave Bert, especially when I couldn't take a turn, and ended in a garden. Bert made the repayments, as all my pay went directly into his account. I got pocket money like Lavender, for girlish essentials and clothes. I accepted it as Anglo-Indian. For Dale's twenty first birthday, I saved up enough pocket money, to buy him a smart Seiko wristwatch, so he wouldn't be ashamed, to take a pulse, on ward rounds, with the consultant and other doctors. The watch had a blue face and silver metal band, and was inscribed with, "I love you". It lasted many years, till it was accidentally "baked", ten years later, put in a low oven to dry the moisture, till I pre-heated the oven for a roast.

The old watch embarrassment, paled in comparison, to Dale and medical students (I referred to as 'Short Coats', as doctors had long white coats), seeing me at work in the pan room, carrying excreta, of all descriptions, in pans, bottles or kidney dishes. The solution, was to hide in the pan room, till all the short coats left. Thanks to my grumbles of messy doctors and medical students, Dale stood out as the only medical student (and later, doctor), to clean up after himself. This endeared him to many a busy nurse. Second and third year nursing students, also gave the first year students a hard time, by leaving them all the tasks, they disliked most. As a people pleaser, I got myself in a mess of trouble, when I became a "Yes" type nurse to all requests. Needless to say, my own performance suffered, and was reflected in a poor ward report as, "disorganisation", till I learned to say, "Yes, if I have time" or "No".

Meantime, the relationship had moved up a notch, with kissing and cuddling, as well as hand-holding, on walks, supposedly to check out the lamp-posts. The foreshore along the Mitchell Freeway, is remembered for shared one dollar burgers (easily the cheapest at the time), from a 'Burger Mobile', set up on the old Canning bridge (where the Freeway once ended, before the extension). Many more homes lined the Swan River. It was at the river's edge, that Dale split his trousers, as he bent down to wash his hands, after 'Fish and chips'. Dale's aunt Maggie (sister of Iris) and uncle Arthur lived in Como, a neighbouring suburb of South Perth. They became surrogate parents, when Lewis dumped seventeen year old Dale, on their door-step, saying he had done all he could for his son. They supported Dale in his final year at John Curtin. Dale was 'Dux' of the school, that year. His name is still listed on their 'Honours Board".

Knitting, first learned during the India-Pakistan wars, from the young wives of junior officers, came in handy, to knit a special birthday vest for Dale. Dale paid me back, for my birthday, eleven days later, by not only learning to knit, but, knitting me a beanie, as a birthday present. I was also able to give Dale another practical gift, more precious than a knitted vest, when I drove us home, whenever Dale got sleepy or tired, particularly at University exam time. Also sorted, was who should pay for our dates, which were simple meals or take-away. We pooled our money, and spent whatever we had, once sharing one burger. I had my pocket money, but, Dale only had what he earned (after buying his medical books), as he gave all his student allowance, in lieu of board. All dates were put on the back burner, for the three month course on, "Early Childhood and Infant Health Nursing" available in Geraldton, Kalgoorlie or Northam (country hospitals).

Northam was chosen, for it's proximity, to Perth, just a three and a half hour drive away. Dale drove to visit on my days off, sometimes for as little as an hour or two, in the nurses quarters, and drove back the same day. It reminded me of boarding school, but, all six nurses had their own rooms, down the corridor, and I was able to get in a lot of dress-making, guitar practice, and letter-writing, which got me through. I also got practice, at deciphering a future doctor's handwriting, which Dale assured me, had been script-like, till he took notes at university. The faster he wrote, the worse it had gotten. I was one of the few, who could read his handwriting. A page of his last letter, in 'Exhibit Four', would attest to this fact. I learned a lot about ear infections and gastroenteritis in children and babies, and my ward report improved. Emails, have replaced letter writing now, but, can't replace the magic of mail, in a letter box.

The only way to spend more time together, was to study together. It was early July, 1975, when Dale came to study with me, for mid-term exams. We had just taken a study break, for ice-creams at the local park, and returned to study at the unit, when "It" happened. We were seated in the lounge, on a two seater couch, facing each other, when Dale began to tell me, what he intended asking Bert and Lavender, of his intentions to marry me. I said, "Never mind them. What will you say to me?" Almost immediately, he asked, "Will you marry me?" Instead of answering the question, I laughingly pointed out, he had not taken the promised, seven deep breaths, before asking. As Dale counted down his breaths on his fingers, I realised it was a serious proposal, and squeaked a "Yes". At twenty one and eighteen, we were on 'cloud nine'. Without any thought of an engagement ring, we rushed to the phone booth, to tell Bert and Iris.

Bert said, we could jump in the lake, for all he cared, and Iris had seen it coming for a long time. Neither of these comments, could burst our bubble, as we bought another ice-cream, and went right back to that park, to swing and celebrate. To pay for the ring, Dale happily went to work, on a building site as a labourer, digging foundations in a rich, hilly suburb, knee-deep in mud, for two weeks. He was so happy, he got off-side with the other workers, for being over-enthusiastic, instead of having more 'smoke-breaks' with them. Dale also got his first ever "Fail", for the test he was supposed to have studied for. He later passed the supplementary exam.

The engagement party, was set for the 16th July, and one aunty, was going to get her long-awaited, revenge. I had laughed to see, Ruby Brady shy away from a public kiss, with her newly engaged beau, at their engagement party. It was my turn to be embarrassed, in like manner, and her turn to laugh, at our engagement party. All the group; Jewels, Elton and Dale's best friend Bob Hope included, finally got to see the diamond solitaire engagement ring. The only family present were Jade, Ruby and their families. Bert had no family in Perth at the time. Some were still in India, while others had emigrated to the U.K. and Eastern States of Australia. The next six months were akin to 'Guns and Roses'.

First the guns came out, in the form of arguments over marriage dates, church and minister. First, Lavender complained, she hadn't in effect, given consent to the marriage. Then she was unhappy, because we had refused to wait, till Dale finished medicine; a three year engagement, instead of two. Dale threatened a pregnancy would ensue, with such a long engagement. Lavender exploded. It just did not sit right with her, for a man (all be it a final year medical student) to be kept by a woman (when she qualified as a nurse). Lavender decided for us, that the wedding would be held, at the family church, in South Perth, as they were paying for it. As Dale and I attended Fremantle, we insisted on Fremantle. Back and forth the arguments went, till beaten down, and stressed over second-year, nursing exams, I capitulated, for I wanted my 'Rainbow' wedding more, than stand by Dale and have a simple one in Fremantle. The date was set for 12 February, 1977 (after I finished).

41

There was a casualty, I failed my second year exams – the first, big, taste of failure. I was summoned to Matron's office, for an explanation. I gave it, and was dismissed, with a stern warning, not to fail my final exams, at the end of third year. I had a lot more riding on this exam, as we depended on my income after the wedding. I was going to have to, draw on my High School study discipline, to make it. Thankfully, third year flew by, mainly because final year students, were no longer 'green-horns'. Also different, was the class of 1/74, chose not to mistreat junior nurses (one stripe on their caps), as was done by third year nurses (three stripes on their cap). Team-nursing came in, as did the caps. The starched aprons, with blue uniforms (with lapels on the sleeve, to denote first second and third year students), was replaced by a blue checked one, with buttons sewn on (instead of buttons like cuff-links, to remove and put on, for each uniform used). The red cape, monogrammed with my name, has since been donated to the hospital museum.

Further changes, were phased in, during the last three months, of third year. The R.P.H nursing, school, was replaced by the, 'West Australian School of Nursing' (W.A.S.O.N). The remaining class of some eighty five students, and the class of 2/74, fought for and got both badges at graduation – both were worn proudly for thirty years of practice, and are treasured mementoes, of a long gone era. Nursing shifted to universities, not long afterwards, as my degree from Curtin attests. It is currently referred to as a "Population Health Faculty", at Curtin. The final third-year exams, consisted of two exams; one in Medicine and the other in Surgery. I have never studied so hard in my life! I redeemed myself, even though these exams, were just ten days before the wedding.

My patients often played a game, of guessing where Nurse Dewar came from, and although they had tried hard over the entire shift, not one guessed, Anglo-Indian. By the time I finished my training, I had it down pat: "I am Indian by birth, of Indian (actually South Asian and East Asian), English (6%), Irish (7%) and a rich European heritage (of many more, thanks to Ancestry

DNA), with a Scottish Surname. If my patients asked me, what nationality I was, the short, answer was "Australian". My nursing classmates, were quick enough, to give me a nickname, but, showed no other interest. One classmate, once called me an "Airhead". South African nurses, were notorious for asking, where I had done my nursing training. One such nurse, reported my work as inadequate, in a bid to have me sacked, so she could replace me, with her friend. The nurse manager found no fault, and dismissed the report. A South African patient, once refused to be cared for, by a coloured nurse.

From time to time, I still get asked where I come from, or there's an assumption, particularly in country towns, where if you are brown, you are automatically considered "Indigenous". I would be proud to be a 'First Australian', if this were true. As it isn't true, I either ask them where they came from, or tell them to stop asking stupid questions, as everyone came from somewhere, even first, second and third generation Australians.

I had to work two weeks extra in lieu of the sick days, to fulfil the three year criteria of the course. This would have taken me, past the wedding date, and delay the honeymoon by two weeks. Dale and I appealed to the Director Of Nursing (D.O.N) for W.A.S.O.N in the new school building, newly built, next door to R.P.H (and no longer in the Administration building of 'Kirkman House'). The price extracted, for the two day exemption required, was a slice of wedding cake, which we remembered to take, as soon as we got back, from our honeymoon. The three years of nursing, ended as it had, for all nurses, who finished before and after me. Mine however, was just before the wedding, after I had worked ten days straight, to make up those sick days missed, to get the wedding day, as days off, at the end. A huge "Roster Request"!

At the end of my last shift, my pen, patient notes, stethoscope, and shoes were gently removed, by all workmates, on morning and afternoon shifts, to make any escape impossible. The "Patient Bath" was prepared with a light-pink, lukewarm, mouth-wash cleansing solution, for the right pre-marriage-eve-send-off. I was marched to it, and dumped in with full uniform and pantihose. A sprinkle of confetti, completed the bath. Shaving cream completed the "hair-do". I squished my way off the ward, to meet Dale and pick up our wedding rings, from the jeweller in Wellington Street. On our way, we discussed who should pay. Then it dawned on us, that it was soon to become, "Our money" and stopped arguing.

It had been a long engagement, with Bert's 'Rules of Engagement'. Bert had insisted Dale brought me home by 10p.m. If we were late, Bert accused me of being a 'slut'. Engaged or not, any 'lap-sitting' was forbidden. So it was prim and proper behaviours, while watching T.V. By this time, Bert had swapped the unit in South Perth, for a big, old, house in Como, closer to aunt Maggie and uncle Arthur, where Dale and I often walked to visit. This was the home I was married from, but, sadly demolished by developers a few years later, when Bert was offered a price he couldn't refuse. With the proceeds, Bert was able to buy two display homes in Bateman; one as an investment in Tarrant Way, the other in Urbahns Crescent to live in. What came next was a "Double Standard".

After banking all my pay, since I began training, as an "Anglo-Indian", Bert insisted I pay for my own wedding outfit, as an "Australian", working student. When I asked him, "How?" I was permitted to keep all of my pay, for the last six months of my training. I asked Lavender, to accompany me, on my wedding, outfit, purchases. I had been looking for it, during my lunch breaks, as it was a short walk down Wellington Street, from R.P.H. I could not decide between a short veil, and a long one, so got both. The six layered veil, bouquet of white roses (the 'roses' part of the guns and roses) and wedding dress, with lots of frills (Dale liked frills), cost me all of the six months pay; $350. I wanted a wedding with an Anglo-Indian flavour.

Lavender kindly made the "Wedding-Favours", of button-hole style roses, carried on cushions, by bridesmaids, to be pinned on all guests. These were also in rainbow theme, to match the bridesmaids, down to the satin covered cushions; two in the shape of 'D' for Dale, and two "E's" for Elizabeth. One cushion was a 'D' and "E', joined together, for the chief bridesmaid Christine. All thanks to Bert who cut the shapes, out of ply-boards, for Lavender to cover. Sadly, Christine never completed her school-leaving year, and went straight into teachers college, ten years later, still on recreational drugs. She remained a drug addict and alcoholic, as a High School teacher. While I had given all my pay, Christine was a 'Hand-out' taker, even when on 90k teachers pay. This legacy was passed on to her son. A double-standard, which nearly cost her son, his life.

Christine wore orange, Vonnie was in green, Ann in lemon (her favourite colour), Blondy in lilac and Gale in pink. All bridesmaids carried a single rose, in their respective colours (also the roses part). The flower-girl wore blue (my favourite), with a matching rose basket of blue roses, for confetti. The groom, best-man (brother Max), grooms-men and page boys (Jade and Ruby's sons) wore neutral beige suits, with matching buttonholes, in theme. There was Bob, Elton, Blondy's finance' Anthony Nelson and an old classmate from John Curtin High. All grooms-men, drove their respective bridesmaids, to church, in their own cars, decorated with the ribbons of the same colour, their bridesmaid wore.

I felt obliged to invite Lizzy (not reciprocated), newly married Sherry (in return for her wedding invitation, three months earlier) and Fergie with friend (as far as I am aware, remains a spinster). As a formality, all aunts and uncles, got formal invitations, as did Lewis Meade, who demanded to be invited with a friend, soon after I had formally met him, for the first time. He attended the service, (seen by Dale, seated at the back of the church) but, not the reception, when we refused (with respect for his ex-wife Iris). Photographs were at the local "Duck pond", where many hours were shared, over the courtship and engagement years.

Although we got an invite to Blondy's wedding a month later, Lavender's prophecy of Blondy, as no more than a 'Social-climber', came true, as soon as her husband, graduated as a doctor, in 1997. Also invited was mature aged, Malaysian student Sue-Lee. She was the only thoughtful one, to drop off a chicken dinner, in case I missed lunch on my busy, special day. By this time, Jewels had won Elton's heart, and were invited as a couple. Jewel's ended with the 'Bridal Bouquet,' and Elton with the 'Garter', the "Australian flavour" to the wedding. Jewels was to give this bouquet away, at her wedding, the following year.

I have never seen a prouder dad, when he walked me down the aisle, and later at the father-of-the-bride, dance with the bride. I was to draw on this memory, years later. After the wedding, Dale called Mr and Mrs Dewar, 'Mum and Dad', and Mr and Mrs Meade, became 'Mum and Dad' to me. Sadly, my parents were to usurp and undermine parental rights, for their own selfish, ends. "Breached Boundaries" in other words, but, to breach them you must have them in the first place. *Boundaries* by doctors Cloud and Townsend recommends ones, "...with a gate to let the good in and keep the bad out..." or "bad things" as Rabi Kushner called it, in his book *When Bad Things Happen to Good People*. And, bad things did happen, when parents did not check out the good **white** doctor's family (as "White was right"). Had they done so, they would've found the Meade family had a bad name in Fremantle at the time.

Iris blamed a 'different culture' for everything; one of the many 'blaming games' played by a majority "People of the lie" as reported by the late psychiatrist Dr. M. S. Peck. Lewis was once heard, asking Dale, what he expected, when he had married a "Wog". Dale's 'closet racism', should have been obvious, by the company he kept i.e. his High School mates (one was a grooms man). Dale once said, "If you knew the real me, you wouldn't like me". But, this closet racism, was to be explained by a 'Traumatised seventeen year old persona', from his parents divorce (after his death). Dale's hypocrisy was finally disclosed at the end of the marriage. No surprise, I got twenty spice sets as wedding presents.

I romantically assumed, Dale was my other half, but, learned years later, from *Rebuilding When Your Relationship Ends* by B. Fisher, two halves only made a quarter. Each partner needs to be a whole, as only one times one, equals one and 100% each is required for 200% input. Married in virginal white, and an exchange of virginity, one to another, was also romantically motivated, a notion from those love story Novels, and far from the painful, awkward reality, in practice. "Dale and friend", were booked at the Astra Lodge, not Dale and the Mrs. We arrived in my car, with confetti spread by the vents, all over us and the car, with 'Just Wed' painted on the rear windshield, and a string of noisy cans, attached to the exhaust.

Uninformed virgins, spelled bruises, and a sleepless night. Armed only with lemonade, in a green bottle, eggs boiled in a kettle, we set off for Augusta and a timber-cabin, booked for a week, followed by a week, in a caravan park in Albany (after deciding not to stay with Dales maternal grandfather), all paid for, with a generous wedding gift, from mum Iris and aunt Maggie. As we fished on the local jetty, we were asked by a by-stander, what we were doing, in such an out-of-the-way place. He smiled when we answered, it was our honeymoon. Ignorance struck again, in the form of "Honey-moon Cystitis"; a urinary, tract, infection (U.T.I). Dale had done a practical session, with the country doctor in town. That doctor smiled saying, "Give it a rest". The practice nurse, admonished the final year medical student, when she saw my bloodied urine specimen. "Didn't you tell your wife, to use the loo after sex?", she demanded. Mount Toolbrinup, in the Stirling Ranges, was christened all the way up and down.

We returned from our honey-moon, to our first home; a one bedroom flat, in Herdsman Parade, Wembley. My first job, as I waited for my Nursing Diploma, was in a local Nursing Home. Sue-Lee now lived with her partner-turned-husband, Allan Bright and their baby son Michael, in the block of two bedroom flats, next door. It felt comforting, to have someone I knew next door. Dale had exchanged the Kombi-van, for a second-hand white Volkswagen, parked alongside my car, in the bay provided, in the car-park, in front of both blocks of flats. Thus began the novel love story, of what can only ever have been, an 'Imitation Love', alongside my nursing career. The next event was unexpected, by accident and not design, hence the aptly captioned chapter to follow.

CHAPTER SIX

Family Planning "Accidentally"

I left the nursing home, as soon as I got the Diploma, and commenced an "In-Service Course" at R.P.H as Sr. Meade. Dale graduated in 1978 and got his first intern-ship, as a Resident, at the Q.E.II Medical Centre (previously Charlie Gardiner Hospital). We intended to leave having a family, for at least a year or two, despite Bert demands, of where the babies were and to stop living in sin. We became a statistic, of the failure of the 'Rhythm method', and use of Condoms as contraception, ten months later, instead of the coveted two to three years. Dale had seen women die, from the (rare) side-effect of clots, by using the "Pill", one a newly-wed. He didn't want us to take the risk, of becoming the one-in-a-million. Once we had had the accident, we saw no reason for birth control, and set out to have a family of six, that Dale wanted.

I ended working full time, until a month before my term date. In so doing, I had created a veritable headache, for administration, as many other pregnant nurses, followed suit, and worked longer, than the six month bench-mark. I was accommodated in the Eye Clinic, in R.P.H. Professor Constable, the head of the Clinic, was compelled to order a 'Baby Delivery Pack'; something he hadn't done for years. He begged me not to put him through that. I still encountered, ignorant racist remarks, from patients in the clinic. The middle-aged man, with a wise grin on his face, asked if there were lions and tigers in my back-yard, where I came from. I retorted, "Just like you have emus and kangaroos in yours", and was rewarded with a sheepish grin, as all the other patients in the waiting room, laughed at him.

The one bedroom unit, was too small now, for our expanding family, so a block was purchased in Spigl Way, Bateman, rather than Booragoon (out of our price range). The plan was to Owner-build, as we wanted several features, from several display homes. While still working full-time, Dale bought an old home and demolished it, for the second-hand Jarrah timber and stock-piled, the machine-cleaned bricks. Heavily pregnant and still working full-time, I went with Dale, only to fall asleep in my car, we named "Buttercup". I re-designed Dale's grand, two-storey plan (this grandiosity, was to re-emerge, eleven years later, for a two-storey, medical centre, with hanging gardens – a grandiosity that was to be connected with Manic Depression), down to a single storey, five bedroom, two bathroom, home. Then Dale cleverly, manoeuvred an open-air 'Atrium' garden, into the middle of the living areas. A reluctant, sceptical (owner-building was in it's infancy), Bank manager, approved the loan to owner-build, after inspecting the second-hand bricks and timber.

Dale began to work on-site, and then go directly to work, sometimes for days on end, without sleep. Concerned, I asked his sister Ann. She simply said, "that's, just, Dale". He had done much the same for his mum's first house, at White Gum Valley, when he re-stumped the back verandah, helped by Max. However, 'that's just Dale' did not cut it, with the brick-layer, sub-contractors. Dale had started crooked brick-work, on every internal wall of the home. Dale sometimes worked over-night, by the light of a gas lamp, even in the pouring rain, propping up collapsing walls. When the brick-layers threatened to walk off the job, Dale compensated them with more pay, and a promise to never touch their walls again. To hide the leans in some walls, all walls were rough-finished, for a "Rustic" look. Still concerned, I asked Iris, and got the same reply. Sleepless nights, were to become a sinister omen, for an equally sinister legacy, that Iris hid, till Dale found out for himself, after having our family.

This house still stands, with it's 'Dale hallmarks' of rough plastered, crooked walls, tongue and groove, solid Jarrah doors and cupboards, solid sleeper, door-jambs, a chimney and fireplace with 'Toodjay stonework', and lots of exposed Jarrah beams and eaves. The 'Postie' did tell Dale to stick to his doctoring, as he struggled to put our mail, in the chunky, Jarrah letter-box. Owner-building netted a substantial saving. On the down side, there was a front and back door, a dirt floor in the en-suite (as plumbers had insisted) and a curtain for privacy, till Dale made all the internal doors, one-by-one.

Jewels had been thrilled at the pregnancy, but dismayed she had to have a second-best friend, Vicky as her 'Matron of honour' instead of me. As it turned out, we never made it to her wedding (also on her birthday). Dressed for the wedding, I bent down to paint my toe-nails. The 'waters' broke and I went into labour. Instead of a wedding, Dale sat me on a towel, and in his heightened state, took the long way around, to the King Edward Memorial Hospital (K.E.M.H), a Public hospital (although we had private cover), just in case an emergency arose for a first baby. With water still running down my legs, we walked to the foyer, where a small child pointed to me and said, "Mummy that lady is doing a wee". This galvanised the staff, to put me in a wheelchair, to take me straight to the delivery room.

I was not in any pain at this stage, but, accepted the apologies, fuss and attention. Joan (for Dale), came into the world, at a quarter past mid-night, and was a text-book, natural birth, except for the cord, around her neck. Present were Dale, both grandmother's and aunty Gale. Elton and Jewels, broke their honeymoon to visit, the next morning, disappointed Joan didn't share her birthday. They relayed the drama of their first night. Elton had somehow managed to set the kitchen alight, at the motel they stayed at. Apart from bruised egos, for running out naked, there was no injury. But it was the look my baby daughter gave me, from her big, dark, velvet, brown eyes, so like my own, that has stayed with me. "So, you are my mum", the look seemed to say. I was to recall this, in sharp contrast, to a new, but, old, family dysfunction, she first took on, as a child of seven, and into adult-hood.

A first baby was a shock, to very young, first time parents. Jewels and Sue-Lee did visit, but, I turned to aunty Jade for advice, for having had both her children, in Australia. I suddenly understood how Jade had felt, from two nuisance teen nieces. The first hint of trouble in my marriage, came when we visited Bert and Lavender (now in Bateman), when Joan was about six months old. After what seemed a minor argument with Dale, he took off across the empty paddock, across from Urbahns Crescent, on the other side of Leach Highway (where S.J.O.G Murdoch Hospital now stands), with me in hot pursuit and baby Joan on my hip. When I lost sight of Dale, I left Joan with her grandparents, and looked for Dale, on a hunch he was with his mum, at her Hilton home (where she moved to from White Gum Valley).

This set up a pattern of behaviour, for the rest of the marriage. With intimacies shared with Iris, (a NO-NO from a Marriage Enrichment Seminar), she became a third partner. Dale turned out to be a 'Mummy's Boy', and no knight in shining armour. Immaturity was a hallmark, of the majority in Dr. M. S. Peck's book. A boy stuck at seventeen, also became, an absent husband, as the surrogate husband of Iris (the "First wife"). He was a pseudo-father to his siblings, to become an absent father and progress to an "Uncle-dad". Dale was to publicly call our children 'Mongrels'. I had not listened, when Lavender said, Dale was tied to his mother's apron strings.

Iris only had eyes for Dale, looking for him, as she brushed past me, and later her grandchildren, just to find and be with my husband, as he cooked at the Bar-B-Q. Dale once told me, he couldn't refuse his mother or tell her 'No'. If he had, she withdrew love from him. This had traumatised Dale, greatly during his childhood; particularly, after the divorce of his parents. His primary family took precedence over our family, every time. On the other hand,

Lavender procured exclusive grandmother rights, when she gave all her attention, to her grandchildren.

Lavender was great for baby-sitting, when I returned to work part-time, at Stirling Hospital. But, this baby-sitting, was to set the stage, for what became "The Other Parents" (a lie), that undermined parents, and brainwashed grandchildren, that resulted with disrespect, and destruction of the mother-child bonds. In hindsight, I lacked *Boundaries* (course and book by Dr. Cloud and Dr. Townsend), and shouldn't have allowed Lavender, to take Joan from me, and comfort her, in my stead.

I learned not to repeat this cruelty, with the mothers of the grandchildren in my life. On the contrary, grandchildren know that mum and dad are the bosses. Being a grandmother is a privilege, not a right, and **adult** children only owe their parents, regard and honour, not obedience, which expires at eighteen. Bert and Lavender, expected obedience, long after Christine and I were adults. Hence a new kind of love, was coined for adult children (estranged ones included), in the sequel. It comes after unconditional love, for children, and tough love for teens. "Just Love" came from an old prophet, who said, "Love without justice is as empty, as justice without love". It is also doing the right, thing ethically speaking (even when no one is watching), as Lavender had written in every greeting card, to her daughters.

I was expecting my second child, when Dale worked all-night-locum's, covering a group of doctors, after hours, while he studied for his 'Surgical Primary Exams', to become an orthopaedic surgeon. Dale passed after three months of study, where some doctors struggled for years, with numerous re-sits. Disaster struck one night, while Dale looked for a house with his torch. Hit on the side of Buttercup, he was propelled into a concrete bus-stop shelter. Buttercup was a wipe-out. With a split lip and fractured ribs, strapped up, he took pain killers, and went back to work, the next day, as I had just given up work. Without private health insurance, we had to return to K.E.M.H for our second baby. Benjamin (Ben) and not Dale junior (as Dale wanted him to be his own man), was born in November, 1980. It was the most painful childbirth, as a face presentation, dry-birth. Years later the damage had to be repaired. Ben wanted to be and did become, taller than his dad at, 6' 3".

We had a 'big little brother' and a 'little big sister' so far, but, Dale wanted six. Looking back, we should've stopped with a pigeon pair. It was recommended to all children thereafter. I had over-ridden my own common-sense, to please Dale i.e. a 'People pleaser' turned 'Husband pleaser'. Dale was now an Orthopaedic Registrar (a pre-requisite for training as an Orthopaedic surgeon), at the Q.E.II Medical Centre. Our next child, was dubbed a "Melbourne baby" for it's conception there. Joan was three, and Ben just turned one, as we flew out, with both children on our laps, for our first holiday to the Eastern States. We planned to stay, at a Motel, when (out of the blue) uncle Grant, invited us, to stay with him in Noble Park. We stayed in their 'Granny flat' at the rear of the home. It was at Luna Park, when on a merry-go-round, with Ben, the morning sickness hit, and suddenly, it wasn't so merry any more.

Also, solved was the mystery of the letter to Harold, that had been unanswered. He never got my letter. Harold's wife Chantelle (from Keti), was expecting their first baby. It was lovely to meet her, and see Harold happily settled. We had not long returned, from the Melbourne trip, when Christine made one of her rare appearances. This is when she confessed, to not posting that letter to Harold. She stayed for awhile, but, did not appreciate, her niece and nephew, waking her up at 5a.m, when she had just gone to bed, after partying all night. When she left, she told our parents, that she had been thrown out. Bert and Lavender believed her, this time and the next, when she complained of me being a 'messy pig', at a short stay, at her Port Hedland home, some twenty two years later.

Dale was now a senior Orthopaedic Registrar, in a second term, still waiting and hoping for that trainee post. He walked out on an operation, when I went into labour. Jacqui (Jacq) was born on Joan's birthday in 1982, also with the cord around her neck. You could say, she was the perfect birthday gift, even though the birthday party was cancelled. As twins, four years apart, they remained close, even after the family fell apart. Dale was not permitted, to care for our children, by Lavender, who had her way with our wedding, then with her brother Grant, forced to put us up in Melbourne, and now had exclusive, grandmother rights. It was to lay the foundation for a lie, that 'Nana raised her grandchildren', not the parents.

When Dale learned an Eastern States doctor (son of an Orthopaedic surgeon), got the trainee-ship, he walked out of his job, without notice, feeling used. But, Dale had told the Consultant, he was wrong, in the middle of a ward round. This was just, never, done and totally out of character. It was the first warning sign, of the dis-inhibition, in the manic phase, of Manic Depression. Had Dale got the trainee-ship, a surgeon would have been a lot more difficult to address than a G.P. Fortuitously, Dale did turn to general practice. Kalgoorlie was Dale's first post, in the Fellowship of Royal Australian College of General Practitioners (F.R.A.C.G.P.).

Kalgoorlie was known as a "Red Light District", so I tagged the family on. Joan slipped on the laundry lino and split open her chin. We went to Daddy's surgery, to have it fixed. Dad sewed it up, while mummy assisted, all whilst Joan screamed "Please don't daddy", next to a waiting room full of people. It didn't help, that Dale's hand shook as he sutured. When mummy covered Joan's eyes, so she wouldn't be scared, she screamed "Don't mummy!" We got dirty looks, as Joan walked out, with red swollen eyes. Unable to rent out Bateman, I went to do night duty, at the local public hospital. When Dale came home to a sleeping wife, with unattended children, he told the doctor to keep his job. Two months later, we went for a family holiday, to India, fully funded and controlled, by Bert and Lavender, and subject to Christine's travel agenda. Thus Jacq's walking was delayed.

The fourth pregnancy, started out with a threatened abortion, at twelve weeks gestation. Its unknown, whether it was pulling a trailer, pushing dirt in a wheel barrow, or the argument with Dale, over cutting a massive century old tree, in his mothers backyard. Local G.P. Dr. Rani was consulted. The due date was close to Ben's birthday, so he ordered a brother. I was having the usual false labour, 'Branxton-Hicks' contractions, so had the birth induced, at Woodside Hospital (no longer exists) by Dr. Rani, on Ben's birthday. Beth, arrived in November, 1984, as an unhappy, birthday present. When Dale brought Joan, Ben and Jacq, to see their new baby sister, Ben cried.

A biggest and smallest, babies were twins four years apart; two sets of twins, four years apart. Beth was the most nervous, clingy, baby out of four, and I got adept, at doing one handed chores, with her on my hip. She barely slept between feeds, day and night. One night, exhausted, I did the unthinkable. I took my baby to bed. Dale turfed mattress, baby and me, out onto the carpeted floor. He was right of course, but, his methods, left a lot to be desired. Suffice to say, I never did it again.

By this time, Jewels and Elton, had three sons, Blondy had two sons and a daughter, and had gone to Pt. Hedland, to work as nurses, with the flying doctor service. Sue-Lee had a daughter and sister for Michael and sister-in-law Ann, had had three children. Grandma Iris supported "poor Ann". Max married Thomasina (we attended with Joan just a month old) and they started their family of three; a pigeon pair and one spare (a son and two daughters). Gale never married and qualified with a double certificate in Nursing and Midwifery.

Dale became a 'Vocationally' registered G.P instead. This is no longer possible, without ten years of post-graduate studies. Dale was again, in the locum G.P after hours service, when he did a 'sit-down locum' for the Deputy head doctor, of the Medical board. When he found a magneto, pulse, machine (used on race horses), being booked for medical appointments, he sent the appointment book, into the "Howard Satler Radio Program".The stealing charge was dismissed, as he hadn't keep the proceeds of the crime. He was re-enstated to the locum service. This doctor also worked at St. Ann's (now Mercy Hospital), my place of employment. When he made the connection, I lost my job.

Not long afterward, Dale was offered a partnership, in a Dr. Weak's practice, after a three month probation. Dale booked a holiday chalet at the Mandurah Holiday Inn. Two weeks short of the trial period, Dr. Weak terminated the partnership, with two weeks pay, in lieu of notice. He couldn't risk Dale, doing what he had done, at the previous sit-down-locum job. We went for the booked holiday. While in Mandurah, Dale spotted an ideal location, to start his own practice, near a Chemist, with a big paved area, in the entire back yard, for parking. The old house, lent itself to be partitioned, for living and consulting. Jewels and Elton, who had shifted to Rockingham, called in to give it a tick of approval.

Bateman was put on the market, and work began, to put a patient toilet into the Mandurah house. We ended accepting a subject offer. To oversee the job, I was alone with four young children, at Mandurah. In Perth, Dale worked full time, in the Locum Service, right through Christmas, and stayed at his fathers place, to catch a break, sleep and save on petrol costs. Dreams generally don't come true, but, mine seemed to sound a warning, that disaster loomed. Dale was the pilot in the dream, and along with the family, crashed the plane. Dale was headed for a break-down, but, insisted on the hour and a half drive, back to see the family he missed. Lewis hit the nail on the head, when he told his son, he had lost his heart.

When he couldn't sleep for nights on end, he self medicated on sedatives. Then his energy levels plummeted. The flat tyre on the car, went unchanged. Self-care was non-existent for days, as he lay lethargically on the floor, staring up at the ceiling, for hours on end. By now, the modifications had been completed. All Dale had to do, was hang out his shingle and start his practice. All the work men had rushed to finish, waiting to see the new doctor in town, particularly as there was a shortage of medical practices. Concerned, I called Iris, who couldn't stay long, as she had to return, to help Ann, with her children. I soon learned, the 'Depression phase', was the only time, Manic Depressives seek help.

Dale booked himself into the Q.E.II Medical Centre, for assessment, and the children and I stayed with Bert and Lavender. Dale was in "Withdrawal" from the sedatives and my dream became a nightmare. It was diagnosed as "Depression", and not just "Reactionary" from overwork, as first believed, but, associated with Manic Depression. Dale spent three months in hospital, and was medicated on mood stabilisers, the effects of which were zombie-like; Dale referred to as "Tardive Dyskinesia" (not unlike shuffling in Parkinsons Disease). Dale once said, the medications felt like, his head was detached from his body. He also hoped, he would never be like Lewis. Sadly, it was to become a self-fulfilling prophecy.

In this foray, Christine decided to marry Patrick, whom she had met in Ferntree Gully, Melbourne. Joan and Jacq were flower-girls, in the red lace and Satan dresses, sewn by me. I wore cream as the Matron-of-Honour, going through the motions, almost in automation, while my mind was else where. Jade and Ruby attended with their respective families. Although Christine looked lovely, Jade asked, where the wedding dress was. The reception was held at Tarrant Way. Christine and Patrick returned to Melbourne, after the wedding. Enter Dr. Meade M.D. For "Manic Depression", and Dr. Jekyll, Heckle and Mr. Hyde (for Hide in depressions).

CHAPTER SEVEN

Dr. Meade M.D. (Manic Depression): Dr. Jekyll, Heckle and Hyde (for Hide)

Borrowed from the cartoon world of Dr. Jekyll and Mr. Hyde, it seemed to fit the real Dale as Dr. Jekyll, Mr. Hyde was for the depressed Dale, that hid, and a manic 'Heckler'. I soon learned, that the main features of both mania and depression, as impressed upon me by Dale's Psychiatrist, Dr. Oberry, were the loss of insight and judgement – the basic tools of a person's cognition, choices and decisions. This wreaked havoc with a Melancholic, Choleric Personality (a 'Sad-Sack', pity-party junkee, in other words). Its been called a "Black Dog". Joan said she had three dads; a real, bad and sad one. Anthony Nelson, on a job with the 'Flying Doctor Service' from Pt. Hedland, called in, to ask after Dale, and our family. Its a treasured memory of care.

When Dale got his energy back, he managed to convince himself, and me, that it had been, just a reactionary depression. No one wants a mental illness label, least of all a doctor, with a high IQ, bordering on genius. Dale was smart enough, to take responsibility, not to father any more children. Dale ignored Iris's objections, that the woman, was responsible. Then Dale asked Iris, which family member, had mental illness. When Iris refused, to give her son the information, Dale legally obtained medical records, and learned of his dad's Heathcote Hospital (now a Restaurant) admission, for a "Personality Disorder". Angry, he asked his mother, why she hadn't disclosed it, before the marriages, of both her sons or advised contraceptives for Ann. Iris simply said, "Because he is your father".

Gale Meade was also diagnosed, with Manic Depression, after she helped herself, to a strangers house. She did disclose abuse, in the children's home, where Lewis had put the three older children, when Iris ran off with baby Ann. Dale was five, and remembered, 'Footsteps coming down the corridor'. Dale had had "Anal dilatation" surgery, when we were newly married. This abused persona was to contribute to the new label to be applied to our youngest daughter in 2008. It was to explain my fifth child.

Dale failed to comply, with the first rule of acceptance, of his diagnosis, as Dr. Oberry (he once called a 'Black bastard', when manic/psychotic) had warned. The second rule, was not to stop taking the mood stabilisers, when he felt good again. For Dale, the highs included racist undertones (when the traumatised teen persona emerged). Insult to injury, Lewis and his brothers, threatened to take me to court. Dale over-rode the court action, in my defence. However, after he learned the Medical Board had been notified (upon my insistence), the blame was re-allocated, to culture and in-law interference. Years later, Dale was to blame me, for his mental illness as, "The Family Problem" (another of Dr. Peck's 'Blaming Games').

Mandurah was sold to Dr. Punyatina. Then one of the cheapest three bedroom, one bathroom homes in Renou Way, Bateman, across the park, from Bert and Lavender, was purchased. It seemed a good idea at the time, needing support, as we did, in the new turn of events. In hindsight, it was too close; another lesson for good boundaries. Dale had signed for this house, while out on leave, without a letter from his treating psychiatrist, to attest to a 'soundness of mind', to sign legal documents. Dale was discharged to Renou Way, not long afterward. As summer approached, Dale began to change, in ways, I hadn't seen before. His speech sped up, and became disjointed, with sentences running into each other, and his sleep pattern altered; going backwards, from shorter nights, to sleepless ones. This I was to learn, was

'Hypo-mania' or 'Pre-Mania', when they are most likely to listen to reason, impossible in psychosis. Dale never listened, also a hallmark of the new label to come.

Dale started to bring home things, to fix, from the rubbish tip e.g. broken wheelbarrows, deck chairs etc. Strewn all over the front and backyard, our home soon looked like, a rubbish dump. With his own brand of reasoning, his speech made perfect sense to Dale, but, no one else, least of all myself. This was the first time (but not the last) I was called a "Stupid bitch" . Dale once said I was not intelligent enough for him. Totally dis-inhibited, unable to keep up the charade, the racist seventeen year old, didn't respect a brown woman, he only tolerated. Those warm, hazel, eyes, turned to black chips, of cold, empty, almost vacant detachment. The abuse turned physical, as coffee mugs and milk cartons, flew across the dining room, to stain the walls and ceilings. "I'm so angry!", Dale shouted.

The first dysfunction, which was to last, way past it's 'due-date', was born in seven year old Joan, as her siblings, then five, three and one, huddled with their protective, big sister, in the main, corridor of Renou Way (when Joan became, 'The Other Mother'). Then the man I trusted and loved, my best friend, confidant and husband, father of our children, pinned me by the neck, against the glass, dining room, sliding doors. I refused to cower, and looked him straight in the eyes. He shouted obscenities and expletives, up-close and personal, to my face.

I had already run around and been given the run-around, and got, "Are you ok?" and, "He is a doctor?". The Q.E.II Medical Centre, finally gave me the answer I needed. A "Form Eleven" (under the 'Mental Health Act' at the time) from a G.P. was required, for admission to Heathcote. I determined to succeed, where Iris had failed to get Lewis help. Lewis had blandly told the police, it was just a 'Domestic Disagreement' which had been resolved. The police officers, had had no way of knowing, of the rages, wife beatings, the knife once held to Iris's throat, or food thrown out of the fridge, and off the table, into the backyard.

I called Dr. Rani, as Dale had recently done a sit-down locum, for her. It was providence when she told me, she had received some complaints from her patients, about Dale's 'inappropriateness'. On the strength of these complaints, and my statements, Dr. Rani filed the 'Form Eleven', for an 'Involuntary Admission' to Heathcote. Four burly policeman turned up, at the door. At 6' 2", Dale was a big bloke. Bert hid in the bushes nearby, and watched Dale go with the cops, as he demanded to be taken to speak to Dr. Rani. I learned later, Dr. Rani had told Dale, through the ambulance window, she was doing this, for his own good. I had taken the children, and fled to Jewel and Elton's place in Rockingham, (Bert and Lavender were too close). Nearly twenty years later, Dr. Rani was to pay a price for this help, when Dale exacted revenge.

This ended being a six month admission. Dale engaged the services of T.D. Hoffsmen and Associates (Dr. Hoff has since returned to private practice), to challenge the 'Form Eleven'. I have since learned, under the Mental Health Act, patients have rights to do so (now called a CTO). Dale also chased six opinions, from surgeons and consultant doctors, he knew. They all said, to take his medications, and he would be okay. As soon as I learned of the legal appointment, I made one for myself. Dr. Hoff called me a "Tough lady", when I refused to let Dale go. Dale did offer me a divorce, which I declined, on premise of an assurance, by Dale's psychiatrist, that Dale could live a normal life, provided he followed the rules. Had I known the true nature of the diagnosis, I would have accepted it, with sole custody (just as Beth's ex-partner did for their son).

Bert did advise divorce, Lavender maintained it was put on, and the Meade's in total denial, blamed culture and in-law interference. Dale relentlessly researched his condition, to find answers. In hindsight, I wished Dale had stayed on that amber light. We attended meetings with the support group A.R.A.F.A.M.I (now 'Helping Hands'), only to find we gave them more information, than we got support, and stopped going after two meetings.

Literature on "Manic Depression" from A.R.A.F.A.M.I., was sent to all family members.

Dale developed all the classic features, of the majority on *The Road Less Travelled,* as reported by psychiatrist, Dr. Peck. Dale was an immature adult, with an inner abused child and a traumatised teen. I became a mum and a dad, in one fell swoop, and dealt with, what was to become chaos, going from disaster to disaster (as Dale called it). I assumed the role of bread-winner, when the sickness benefits, were insufficient, and took on full-time work, as a 'Silver Chain' community nurse. This would have been far better, as a divorced mum of four (with sole protective custody). Dr. Phil McGraw of the *Dr. Phil Show* often says, "Better to be from a home of abuse, than in one".

Based on the prognosis for Manic Depression, upon Dale's discharge from Heathcote, not wanting him to go cap in hand for a job, and a mental illness in the other, a sole-medical-practice was considered, the best way to earn, for our young family. This would have been a non-entity, in the case of the fore mentioned divorce. More than likely, Dale would've been under a Guardianship and the office of the Public Advocate (OPA), with a Disability Support Pension (DSP), in long or short term, supported living. Two blocks were procured from 'Homes West' (Welfare housing, now 'Department of Communities'). 'Location, location, location", Dale had chanted, was the key to success. I enrolled in TAFE, to learn typing and basic computer skills. However, nothing prepared me for the opposite pole to mania; i.e. an equally deep, depression. With sleep disturbance, in common, there was a high risk of 'self-harm'. Dr. Peck warned, that some of the majority, do get in touch with their inner reality, can't handle it, and suicide. Self-harm is a distinct feature of the new label. Dale once told me, he swallowed weed killer, and tried to gas himself, in his car, with a hose pipe. Lucky the hose pipe leaked.

Oblivious to this danger, I accepted a coffee invitation, with a bunch of girls, after typing class. I came home, to find my entry, barred by a Dr. Smith from Dr. Hong's (now retired) surgery (where Dale had worked for a short while). Dale had meticulously dissected out, the Radial and Ulnar arteries in both wrists, medical-student-style. His saving grace was, that he was right-handed, and not as good, dissecting left-handed. Pre-meditated with precision, he made sure I wouldn't come home to the, "dead person in a blood-bath, scenario" and called Dr. Hong. He also made sure the children were with their grandparents.

Dr. Smith was supposed to have pronounced him dead, and been there for me. Dr. Smith managed to clean the smeared blood, all along the corridor, and around the bath, and bandage both wrists, by the time I opened the front door. Some of the evidence remained, but, I only had eyes, for the man I had almost lost forever. I followed the Ambulance to the Q.E.II Medical Centre, for plastic surgery on both wrists. The resident on duty, in the casualty department (now E.D), looked sadly at me, as he said Dale would succeed one day, and that there was nothing I could do, to prevent it. He was to be proved right, a few years later. When blood loss confusion, was mistaken for mania, I stepped in and demanded his haemoglobin results. Two units of blood were ordered instead, without apology. Depressants, would've driven him into an even deeper depression. I was surprised to learn, Thomasina and Iris came to visit Dale in hospital. They never called me.

Although believed at first, to be because of guilt at passing on the illness to our children, it was actually the guilt, for adultery with prostitutes, his psychiatrist had strongly advised against ever revealing. As part of the increased libido in mania, it was best left alone. But, the marriage had lost it's 'Innocence'. He was to disclose it five years later. He was angry at Iris and rightly so, because all ten grandchildren stood to inherit it. Thomasina dismissed it, out of hand. Her eldest son ended with a diagnosis of depression, and Ann's eldest, with Bipolar Disorder (as far as is known). I was angry at the choices taken away from our family.

We all "Walked on egg-shells". I even gave in to pay off Iris's mortgage, just to keep the peace. Enter "Passive Aggression" in the form of 'Retail Therapy' (just like Lavender). It began with a stereo, grandfather clock, Royal Doulton Dinnerware and gold cutlery. Later designer clothes and holidays we couldn't afford, followed, to sublimate some of the pain. It was when I learned the bank loan for plant and equipment for the practice, had been used for prostitutes. Angry, I ignored Dale's repeated requests, for an emergency fund, which was never saved. Worse still I went along with his manic spending. We went backwards, every time Dale had to go to hospital, as overheads had to be paid, even when not working, and later, the share of overheads, allocated to each associate, of the practice. Since then, I have learned, to make money work for me, rather than work for it, mind my own business and own the real estate under the business, from *Rich Dad, Poor Dad*, by R.T. Kiyosaki, basically, good stewardship or money management, which stood Eagles in good stead, when they retired.

While Dale was recovering in hospital, the two blocks, from Homes West, were approved for a medical centre. With Dale in hospital, a bank loan was out of the question, so I asked Bert. Bert demanded, the blocks be purchased, in his name. I had no other option, but, to accept, as I had been raised to respect, honour and obey. I have since learned, that obedience expires, at eighteen, but, not respect and honour. The cheapest three bedroom, "Homes-West" house, with some minor alterations, was built on the blocks, to be used as a 'Doctor's surgery', without any consultation with Dale.

Dale was provisionally registered with the Medical Board, on the proviso of regular, monthly, reports, from his treating psychiatrist, Dr. Clayton, to attest, to his fitness to practice. Dale started the practice, after his discharge from hospital. It was a 7a.m to 7p.m 'Bulk-Billing', practice, with Dale doing his own after-hours calls, as we couldn't afford the fees, for the locum service. Bert and Lavender, also had full control of the children. Grandparents had already told the children, that daddy was mad, and mummy didn't know what she was talking about. This set the ground rules for the parent take over, by the 'Other Parents' and a legacy of lies, which began with 'Nana raised the grandchildren'.

As a direct result, the first father of lies was birthed, together with disrespect for parents. It lay dormant till the children were adults.

However, I was in my element as a nurse-receptionist-cleaner-gardener – 'A Jill of all trades", and when it became a medical centre, with seven units, also a 'Strata Manager'. Bert regularly attended, resplendent in Bush-shirt, shorts and thongs, as "Practice Owner", as he often announced to all the waiting patients, in the small lounge area, used as a waiting area. Bert used mattress tape, from his factory, for a fence, the Cockburn Shire, duly demanded to be removed. He never understood, only a doctor could own a practice, and he only owned the building.

When the numbers had grown to a hundred a week, Bert was asked for a formal lease. He demanded one third, of the gross income, and came to check the books. Thanks to Dales misuse of the bank loan, most of the income, was regularly poured, into medical equipment, as we lived on a single, meagre, wage. After six months, the rent was seven times the average, for a medical premises. Often told off for being late, when our children said we loved the surgery more than them, I went to do battle with Bert, to reclaim our surgery and children. After a heated argument, and after consultation with Christine, about the "Family Business", Bert decided to sell it back, at a profit of $25,000. He smirked, believing no bank would lend, to a mentally ill doctor. I learned later, that Christine had suggested a much larger profit margin. We did not speak to Bert and Lavender for two years, till Dale insisted we apologise (for being right?), setting yet another bad precedence. Dale hadn't wanted the children to miss out on their grandparents.

We employed our first receptionist, Margaret. Margaret (and all future receptionists), and later associate doctors, got the A.R.A.F.A.M.I. literature on "Manic Depression", to support Dale. The South Lake Surgery, was extended to include, units for a chemist, dentist, physiotherapist and optometrist, as the Jandakot Medical Centre, all pre-sold from plans, to these professionals, who gave the builder, their respective internal plans. A car park was constructed in front of these units. Renou Way was sold, and the house next door to the medical centre was purchased. We lived in the three bedroom, one bath home, for the shortest time, as realisation dawned, of why doctors, don't live next door, to their practices.

We soon had patients, waiting to see Dale, in the lounge and dining room, waving to the kids, as we finished our evening meal. This and a house fire, accidentally lit by three year old Beth, playing with matches, decided the purchase, of a five by two home, in Anscombe Loop, West Leeming, near the local primary and high schools. The house next door to the centre, was then partitioned, and sold to a podiatrist and dental technician. This seven unit, medical centre, at the corner of Berrigan Drive and Forrest Road, now stands as a monument, to our achievement. Dale had a twenty minute drive, via the new Kwinana Freeway extension, and the Berrigan Drive exit.

The children continued to go to Bateman Primary. Beth refused to attend a four-year-old, Kindergarten, and became even more clingy. She managed Bateman Pre-primary, the following year. She became spoiled, as well as clingy, when, as the only one to shop with mum, she got whatever she asked for, be it toy or story book, much to the chagrin, of her older siblings. I had just created my own spoiled brat. It was to take a whole lot of tough love, and two weeks, to take back my "No", some eleven years later. With a November birthday, Ben started behind the eight ball with his reading and needed extra classes, when he began school. He was a big boy, but, still got bullied for being 'slow' in reading.

After I reported it, to the principal, and named the bullies, it stopped. Ben found a good friend, in Adam, who defended Ben, and took him tadpole hunting, at a local pond. Then Ben caught up his reading, and this problem ceased. Jacq as a Meade, became daddy's pet, jealous Joan and Ben began to beat on Jacq, while waiting for me (mostly late), to pick them up, after school. Other parents had observed the beating, and alerted me to it. Jacq's little legs were bruised. I was on time for pick-ups thereafter. When Beth got to first year, we were in West Leeming, so all four children, finished the year at Bateman Primary i.e. years one, three, five and seven.

Ben, Jacq and Beth went to West Leeming Primary, the following year. Joan was not looking forward to Leeming High, as all her friends were going to Rossmoyne or Willeton. Joan overcame her lonely first days, by heeding my advice, to take a book to school everyday, and read at recess breaks. Not only was it to engender, a love of reading and literature, taking the literature prize when she graduated from the high school, but, she found a best friend for life. Shirley Watsonia, was the only inquisitive one, to ask Joan, what she was reading. Ben also found, long term friends, at this high school, namely Hans Woolfram, and Sunil Shah. Jacq met her long term friend Candice Bergman (Candy) at the primary school, and Beth had Elaine Jungle, whom she went to gymnastics with, and both were awarded many trophies and medals.

About five years after Dale's suicide attempt, I instinctively sensed a growing, barrier, between us. I forced a confession, out of Dale, forgiving him, before he told me. Dale begged on his knees and pleaded for me to let it go, as the prostitutes had been mania-driven, by astronomic libido. When I asked Dale, how many women there had been, he answered too many to count. The first reaction was to take a shower, to wash away, all those women. The second was to get tested by a G.P. I didn't know, for STD's. Thomasina said I had not given Dale enough, and Iris said nothing. Bert had confronted Dale and in the fight, Dale broke Bert's glasses. Lavender was to tell our children not long after, when the children asked us, what a prostitute was. Another control measure was 'Anorexia Nervosa', to make myself perfectly beautiful, so Dale wouldn't stray again.

Guilty if I missed, even a day of the seven-day aerobics ritual, followed by an hours circuit with weights, the kilos fell away. Some of the diet was healthy, drawing from my knowledge, as a nurse. But some, like just a lettuce leaf, for a meal, left a lot to be desired. All I could see, was my thin face in the small mirror, and a six pack on my flat chest. Jewels joined me in dieting at first, but, couldn't keep up. It was when she asked me, to try on a dress, that was a size too small for her, that I first saw myself, in her full length mirror. With my prominent rib-cage, I looked like, one of those starving millions, in an African famine, so often seen in the media. I had dropped thirty kilos. The weights circuit was dropped, and aerobic sessions reduced to three a week. I regained my minimum weight. Needless to say, the gut had taken a beating and was to pay for accumulative stress at forty and then sixty. First with Irritable Bowel Syndrome (IBS), followed by a paralysed gut, with multiple food intolerances, overcome or managed by medications and diet.

The children took to calling Dad an "Uncle-Dad", when he showed more interest in his nieces and nephews. According to a course on 'Family of Origin', the first man in a daughters life, is her dad, and the first woman for a son, is his mum. An absent dad, and a not all there mum (playing Mr. Dad), led to promiscuity of all children, looking for love in their relationships, to a greater or lesser degree; from four serious relationships to multiple marriages, one-night stands and prostitution. Although no family (except Bert, Lavender and Iris), showed up at birthday parties, on the flimsy excuse of no formal invitation, we were expected to go, for their birthday parties, as "Family", without a formal invite.

Although Joan had already said, to get a divorce, just aged eleven, it came two years later, when I was finally able to share, Dale's adultery, with Christine and Patrick. They had just moved back to Perth for good, with their two year old son, William (Will). Christine said to leave my unfaithful husband. Still hurting, I took the children, then seven, nine, eleven and thirteen to stay with my sister. A divorce lawyer was appointed, and papers served on Dale. Dale was frantic as Lewis had just passed away, and began to stalk Beth at her primary school. When the judge refused sole custody, citing fathers rights (in the media at the time), the divorce was cancelled. When I got back to West Leeming, I learned Max, was the executive of Lewis's Will, not Gale or Dale. I returned home, to protect my children till they were adults. Patrick exacted revenge, and stole the money I had put in his account, for safe-keeping. Again, Bert and Lavender said and did nothing.

At this time, Bert and Lavender had been in an argument for two weeks, about giving Tarrant Way, to Christine, as an early inheritance. Urbahns Crescent, was supposedly my inheritance. Bert had resisted, at first, demanding a DNA test. Although the test was never done, Bert suddenly capitulated, and transferred the house. She lost it to her tenants, two years later, in lieu of monies owed to them. She moved to Pt. Hedland, as a fully qualified, High School teacher. This event, came back to haunt me, with a 'Secret Lie', that had been taken to the grave, by Lavender, Christine and Bert. Ancestry DNA done after their deaths, for interest, was to shed light on this lie, and is discussed in the chapter on 'Weddings, Funerals, Deaths and Births'.

Beth was only seven, when Dale first beat her, for not sleeping, in her own bedroom. Beth had taken to coming with her doona, to sleep on our bedroom carpet, holding my hand. The corridor lights were on as usual. This had begun, with a bedside light, since Joan had cried in her cot, and only went back to sleep, when she knew, mum was where the the light was. This wasn't enough for insecure Beth. Then Dale locked her out in the dark, to 'get over her fears of the dark'. Asleep I hadn't heard her, but, Joan did, and let the terrified Beth back in. This was to mark Beth for life, as an abused child persona (as had the abuse of Dale at five, in that children's home).

Ben had also gotten a beating, for coming out of his big-boy bed, for the first time. After singing several lullabies, about every animal possible, going to sleep, he emerged wide awake six times, to peep at us, watching T.V in the family room, at Spigl Way, Bateman. He got a strapping too, just as Dale had been belted by Lewis; a 'Family of Origin' punishment, also for telling lies. There were to be other belting's, for Beth and

Ben, on bare bottoms, that left bruises. Although I had cringed at the memories, as I had been beaten, I accepted it as a father's discipline, and also a 'Family of Origin' punishment, for being 'bad' and making me smart. I said and did nothing, just like Lavender. I have since learned, it is child abuse, and done to humiliate, and in anger not love (and in my case, also the victim of pedophiles).

After numerous holidays, to save the flagging friendship, especially since she acquired, new friends (who were first generation Australians), going to Bali with Jewels, I pushed in to join the party. Dale begged me not to go, but, I needed my 'Holiday Fix". Not only was it a miserable holiday, as all the kids got 'Bali-belly', but, as a tag-on, the children and I, were in a different motel, a good walk away, up the beach. Worst of all, Jewel's mum, and I ended in a fight, over a pack of cheap socks, because I was leaving the next day, while they remained for another week, and could easily have gotten the next bundle. I refused to back down (as a migrant). I was to pay a higher price, for the holiday. Dale burned all twenty family, photo, albums, in the heat-form fireplace, except for the wedding album. The only photographs, of that time, were the ones given to grandparents, taken at birthday parties. This was to give credence to the lie that, 'Nana raised her grandchildren', by Joan (fifteen at the time), who once said, "Photographs don't lie".

Dale brought home a kitten we named "Boots" for her black paws, and bought a golden retriever pup we named "Nala". Joan couldn't abide, the puppy noises, while she was studying, for her school leaving exams, and left home, much as aunty Gale had done, also at sixteen. So, I was to miss some of her precious teen years, given to the Watsonia family instead. I am grateful, that while I missed her sixteenth birthday party (at the Watsonia's with, her favourite Black Forrest cake, I provided), I did not miss out on her high school ball, or choosing her ball gown. I met her first boyfriend, a law student named Clarke Kent. He gave her a beautiful corsage, after Thomasina did her hair.

Joan moved into her own place, after enrolling in a double major, in psychology and law, at Murdoch university. To supplement her student allowance, she worked part-time, with a reference from her high school, literature, teacher, as a PCA (patient care assistant) at the newly built S.J.O.G. Murdoch hospital. I looked forward to Joan and Shirley, popping in, to raid the fridge, on their lunch breaks or after work. Two years later, Clarke dumped Joan, as an inconvenience, when he went to Sydney, to do his "Articles", devastating Joan, as she intended to transfer her law degree, to Sydney, to go with him. She returned home, to heal at eighteen.

Not long afterward, the Nelsons returned from Pt. Hedland, for Anthony to do medicine. Dale put the expensive medical texts, through the practice accounts. Blondy worked night duty, for six years, to put her husband through, medical school. In return, Anthony helped set up the fortieth, surprise birthday party for Dale. After the party, Dale begged, me never to do a surprise birthday party, again. I never did. A holiday to the 'Gold Coast' was organised as a birthday present. While we were in Queensland, the Anorexia Nervosa, exacted it's price (I.B.S.), diagnosed at the Brisbane public hospital. Cumulative stress had taken its toll, also, I had returned to some university units, to convert my R.P.H. Diploma into a degree, at Curtin University.

Dale in turn, threw me a 'Mad-Hatter' party, for my fortieth, three years later. Blondy and Anthony did attend. This is when Blondy slapped Ben, when he called her a "Stupid cow". It was my place, as his mum not hers, and it soured the friendship, which ended, after we went for Dr. Nelson's university graduation. Dr Nelson became director of the Armadale Hospital, where Sue-Lee, worked as a nurse practitioner, in the renal unit. After his graduation, we only got greeting cards, with 'Dr. and Mrs Nelson' printed on a gold label. Blondy had her social status, and didn't need a mentally ill doctor any more. There ended, the one-sided friendship.

My fortieth birthday gift, was a trip to India; a North Indian holiday, to Delhi and Secunderabad. Dale struggled with the culture shock, and disturbed sleep patterns, from different time zones, but, never complained. I was his "Indian princess". We based ourselves, at Madras/Chennai, where the plane first landed, and where best friend June's, youngest sister, and husband, lived. As a thank you, we gave them a deposit for a flat. For the first time, we asked Iris to babysit. Lavender's objections were side-lined, to give Iris a chance, to re-connect, with her grandchildren. She ended up doing more than just baby-sitting. When Beth brought home, a Ouija Board, she told Beth to take it right back.

Dale had been in practice, for ten years, when he lost his psychiatrist. It is a testament to the late Dr. Clayton's good care, that Dale was able to practice as a G.P. Dr. Clayton once hospitalised Dale, for ten days, at the mental health clinic at S.J.O.G. Hospital, Subiaco (it no longer exists). I believe the death was the catalyst to the instability and events that followed, in its wake. Dale was hard pressed, to find a replacement. A paediatric psychiatrist, agreed to take over Dale's care. The problems began immediately, with contraindicated medication, prescribed for Dale, who began popping these pills like 'Smarties'. It made Dale psychotic over-night.

He had used up the entire prescription, when swaying and lurching, with slurred speech, he demanded his car keys. When I refused, he began smashing things in the house. The floor was soon littered, with broken glass, from a smashed T.V. Wedding presents and crystal glassware, given by the late Lewis, soon joined the T.V. I stopped Dale, when he got to Ben's precious computer, with his favourite Commando game. Ben was seventeen, the same age as Dale had been, when he defended Iris. Ben defended me, by hitting his dad, with his cricket bat, as hard as he could, to no avail. Jacq was helping Ben and shouted to Beth, to call 000. Ben begged me, to give his dad, the keys. I called Iris and Max. "All I wanted were my car keys", pouted Dale to his mother, brother and the police, that turned up. Luckily, the police believed Beth.

Dale had pushed me backwards, and I had fallen, onto a bookcase on the floor. I sustained a Haematoma (blood blister), in my lower lumbar spine. I suspect this injury, was to be the precursor, to the total and permanent disability, I was to retire with, after thirty years of nursing. In my nightgown at the time, I showed the injury to the cops. The bruises came out the next day, and my G.P. gasped when he saw them. Neither Max nor Iris asked after me or the children, they had eyes only for Dale.

Dale was taken, to the lock-up, ward at Alma Street, in Fremantle Hospital (F.H). The paediatrician and his secretary, distanced the practice, and themselves, from what had occurred, and blocked my calls. I lost my job, when I told them, about the domestic violence, and back injury. Dale was now re-diagnosed, with the sever type two, renamed "Bipolar Disorder", which Dale also began to research, by reading articles. He tried the herbs recommended. I learned much from these articles. This time, Dale nearly killed me, because of a wrong medication, with amnesia of the event, besides. I was doubly traumatised, when I retold the events, in Alma Street, a week later.

By this time, Dale's associates, had had enough of covering, for Dale's episodes, over the entire association, and threatened to walk out. Dale had not listened to take time off, either. As soon as Dale was discharged, he discussed dissolving the association, and organised the sale of the practice to his associates, and their respective family trusts. Dale did not want to destroy it, any more. He walked away and decided to swap roles. I became Mrs Dad and he was Mr Mum. I got a full time job in hospitals, chasing speciality fields, I was interested in, such as cardiology and orthopaedics. Mr Mum got a part-time job, doing medicals, for migrants and army recruits.

Joan met Ryan Big, another Murdoch university, psychology student, not long after Clarke had dumped her. Ryan began to stay with Joan, in the games room, just over weekends. There were the seven of us and a cat, dog, and budgie for Ben, named "Earl".

74

Ben had been transferred, to All Saints College, in year eleven, without discussion, when he went for a holiday in Adelaide, to visit a friend, who had just moved there. Ben paid for his trip, with earnings from KFC. Ben rightly resented not being asked or told. When we offered, to transfer him back, to Leeming High, he decided to stay, especially when he was joined, by his friend Sunil Shah. The dress code and school name, were to give them the edge into, Curtin university, to do Pharmacy (Ben) and Law.

Jacq met Ryan Little, so that 'twins', were both going out, with a big and little Ryan. When 'Big Ryan' began to stay all week, they were asked to move out, by Mr. Mum. Joan and Ryan got a rental duplex in Shelley. I passed the Mature Age Entrance Exam (M.A.E.E), and applied to do medicine. I was thirty-nine, and out of more than five hundred applications, I was one of twenty, selected for interview. I was one of three, who missed out, on seventeen places, at UWA. The letters still sit on file, along with my degrees.

This was final closure, although I did try, another application, the following year, without response. I fast paced the remaining units, in my degree, and graduated at forty, with a BA Sc and went on to do a Masters in orthopaedics. The whole family, proudly came to my graduation, and a photograph to mark the occasion, was given to Bert and Lavender, along with a copy of the Degree, to hang on their wall, beside Christine's High School Teachers Degree, in their family room. I had also proudly attended Christine's graduation. So much for being the stupid one, and Christine was beautiful.

It was July, and as usual, Dale threatened to leave. But, this time, he followed through. I asked him to go to hospital. Then Dale lied (another of Dr. Peck's majority of the lie, hallmarks) and promptly turned this request to go to hospital, into a demand at first, then followed by a "Liz kicked him out", to his family and all friends, who accepted without question. No one ever called the well partner, to check on the facts. Bert who was present at the time, also asked Dale to get help. Dale took some clothes, and went to the Raffles Motel (remodelled since then) at $100 a night. This time Dale was hospitalised, when he attended his appointment at Alma Street.

When the 'Men's Home' refused to take Dale, a unit was rented in South Perth, for Dale's discharge. This first separation traumatised Beth, who at thirteen had just begun high school, and to a lesser extent, Jacq at fifteen, both blamed themselves, for their Dad's departure, from the marriage and family, as children do in separations and divorces according to Rev. A. De Visser, in *Healing For Damaged Emotions* (First Draft). Jacq turned to Marijuana for solace and led Beth into it. Feeling unwanted, since little, Jacq also disclosed teen depression, and needed a specialist. Drug free Behaviour Modification Therapy (BMT) helped, but, not as much as the apology from Joan and Ben, for those beatings at Bateman Primary. Although Jacq was able to move on, Beth got stuck as a traumatised teen, (just like Dale at seventeen), and turned to drugs, as a problem-solver, ever since.

Then the Dewar pride, deserted a 'North Indian princess', who begged Dale to reconcile, kneeling in a public car park, in a local Bullcreek shopping centre. When he refused, the wedding ring was thrown at him, only to beg for it back. The 'Butterfly' had morphed into a 'Turkey', as she circled "...a mountain of doom", as described by B. Fisher, in *Rebuilding When Your Relationship Ends*. Joan once said, two "Fruit-loops" couldn't live together, neither could two Turkeys. One Turkey was "Responsible for" his single mother and sisters; "His three girls", instead of 'Responsible to' his three daughters (*Boundaries* by Dr. Cloud and Dr. Townsend). This separation, was the beginning of the end, for the marriage.

CHAPTER EIGHT

The Beginning Of The End

This seven year period constituted, a five year separation and two year reconciliation. I suspect to soften the blow, Dale suggested living apart, working together, for the common good of all, in our unique set of circumstances. A first (of two) settlement was done, to protect family finances, from Dale. The Leeming home was for the family, and Dale purchased a one bedroom, one bath, flat in Victoria Park, affectionately nickname, "The Hut", as I had once said, I would live anywhere with Dale, even a humble, hut. However, this set the stage, for being neither single, nor married. The youngest two, already felt abandoned, but, when Dale played games with their child support, it re-enforced the abandonment. I went into automation: eat, sleep, work. It gave me little time to think. I was headed for my first "Burn out", after three months.

This is when, Jacq and Beth turned to drugs for solace, and hid it for a year. The first I knew, was when I was summoned to the school office, by the Principle of Leeming High School. In full-time work, I had missed the tell-tale signs of drug use, right in front of me. Apparently twenty children were playing truant, in the large, shed in my backyard. Then I made a startling discovery, in my shed, that Christine informed me, was a "Bong". Both my youngest daughters, were not just smokers, but, "pot-heads", that turned into a long term addiction for Beth. Unlike Jacq, Beth was to proceed to harder drugs. Ben turned to alcohol for solace. There were many holes, punched by a drunk angry Ben, on the internal doors, of Anscombe Loop, Leeming. Before the year was out, Leeming was sold, in favour of two units in Shelley, close to Joan and Ryan, and a four by two, new home, on a block in Bibra Lake. Ben refused to live at Bibra Lake, as he considered the suburb, below standard.

Ben moved into the main bedroom, of one of my Shelley units, rent-free. Hans Woolfram, took the second bedroom, for half the rent. Ben also kept both; his student allowance and rent assistance, from Centrelink. A newly separated, American-born, New Zealand (NZ) and Australian nationalised, woman named, Crystal or Crys, rented the other Shelley unit next door (when Joan refused to rent it). At the same time, nursing was exchanged, for a four day job, in the city, for HIH Insurance, as a "Medical Case Coordinator". Loneliness drove both women together, at weekends, sometimes going to the Burswood Casino. Ben would pop in, on study breaks, or for a meal. Crys was a great cook. I had been at HIH about a year, when Beth got herself diagnosed, as ADHD, by using her picture-perfect memory, to memorise the symptoms for the G.P., consult. She began to sell the Amphetamines at school. Dale tried but failed to stop the Scripts. Beth in effect, had a brake and accelerator, at the same time. Then Beth almost got raped and murdered, by getting into a car, with strangers, to get drugs. "Panic attacks" followed.

Despite my pleas, not to kill my daughter, Lavender took Beth, to drug dealers, any hour of the day or night, believing she was keeping her safe. Once, Lavender brought Beth, to my work place, only to steal my purse. I tried to have her charged, but, she was too young. Already in the early stages of Dementia, all pleas fell on Lavender's deaf ears. I was well advised, by a family lawyer, to save everyone else in the family, by isolating the drug problem. Bert came to the park and ride, to tell me, it would be better, if I got a job transfer. I had to take Beth away, from drug dealers, as well as her enabling grandmother. At sixteen, this was being 'Responsible to and for' Beth (*Boundaries Course, Boundaries* by Dr.'s Cloud and Townsend). Parents are only 'Responsible to' adult children (not for). I got a job transfer, to HIH Melbourne, as a 'Claims officer' (the only one available at the time). For some unknown reason, Bert and Lavender, changed it into a trip to see Harold.

Hans left, when I wouldn't reduce his rent, for a smaller room. No surprise, the Woolfram family distanced themselves,without empathy for a single, working mother (after a unilateral visit from Dale no doubt). Jacq was moved in with her brother, as she continued at SAE Sound Technician College. She had tried Radio Academy, but, didn't like it. Both courses had cost $10,000. Elton and Jewels separated, and Elton rented Bibra Lake, when I left. My only solace, as I left, was that Joan and Ryan were nearby and motherly Crys was next door. Ben, Jacq and Crys saw us off at the airport. Beth had been warned, not to use street drugs, as they could contain a rat poison base. A new colleague (not uncle Grant), helped find a two bedroom unit in Hawthorn, close to work and the city (by tram). After a two week orientation, I got thrown into the deep end.

To clear the three month back-log, although I worked sixteen hour days, Monday to Saturday, I couldn't make a dent in the pile. At this time, an ambulance had to be called, with police escort, when Beth went into "Withdrawal", locked herself in her bedroom, and began self-mutilating with a knife (the very first 'Self-harm' of many to come). The police chased her down the street, when she got out the window. Assessed at hospital, she was not diagnosed with Bipolar Disorder (missed opportunity), despite family history. Beth did settle after this episode.

Beth was on her medication for ADHD and natural remedies, when enrolled in Hawthorn High school. Best of all, after holding my "No", for two weeks, Beth gave it back. All went well, till the gangs asked Beth to join. When she refused, they ostracised her, and gave her a hard time. It was a stabbing of a student, at the bus-stop, where Beth waited for her bus, that was her undoing. Unfortunately, it had also been a case of mistaken identity. Beth refused to go to school. A private school was not an option, as term had already started. Instead of staying home alone, Beth came to the office to help, even on Saturday, she said to protect me, in the late evening, tram rides home. This was the very first time, Beth couldn't be alone, and because of it, was to end up homeless, after she destroyed a serious relationship. The job wasn't working out, so I looked for a job in nursing.

In February, Dale rang at work to wish me for our wedding anniversary. Tired, I rebuffed him with it being just another day. Then Dale sent divorce papers, with a book on *Rebuilding When Your Relationship Ends* by Dr. Cloud and Dr. Townsend (a reference in this book). Everyone in the Mailing room, was privy, to my private documents and book. Dale cried, as he told a new friend of his (my Eagle), that his wife, had 'kicked him out, and run off to Melbourne' (a lie for sympathy). The Divorce was booked for May. So much for living apart, staying married, for the common good of the family. Looking back, I can see a devious, plan unfolding, that had been a long time coming. Whatever Dale said and did from here on, spelled 'Divorce'.

After three months, it wasn't IBS or burnout, but, chest pains, which sounding the alarm, this time. An E.C.G (electrocardiograph) didn't show any changes, but, I decided to resign, and look for a job transfer, back to HIH Perth, but, there were only part-time jobs available. So, the Removal Company, was paid another $10,000, to take all the furniture, and car, back to Perth. I had borrowed to finish the Bibra Lake Home, now Removal-Van costs and Beth's private school fees, from Bert, and owed, the princely sum of $55,000. Beth had to catch up on a terms work, and set her heart on medicine. I was short on rental income, from Crys, every time Ben asked her for money. Ben never knew, it came out of Crys's rent. There was no rent from Elton, as he had moved out, and moved on, in a new relationship. Harold came by, to help pack up the push-bikes, for the plane trip back to Perth.

I had a unique chance to say goodbye, to my first love, nearly thirty years after we said, "Farewell". For just a moment, I was fifteen and Harold sixteen, as we kissed a bitter-sweet, innocent and honourable, 'Good-bye'. Another Hawk-Dewar love story bit the dust, and that prophecy by a neighbour, had borne out. I had chosen looks, over heart, and been very miserable. Before he went into a coma, Lewis advised to never have regrets. I grieved what could have been. When Bert and Lavender, made the Melbourne trip, about chasing Harold, it ended up on the Podanur Gossip-vine, as a sordid affair, with a married man. I wrote to his wife to explain, and assured her, it was just a 'Goodbye'. I didn't care what people said. I knew the truth or facts. There is little doubt, that this gossip, eventually reached uncle Grant, his wife and her family, and made waves on my FB.

Beth and I returned to Perth in April, and Crys gave us a lift back to Bibra Lake. Jacq came back to Bibra Lake. Then, either because of her addiction, she forgot or wilfully lied, (with motive to use, for her own end, as 'People of the lie' do) that she had no home to go to. The fact is, she did have a home, and had not been abandoned, staying with her brother when I took Beth to Melbourne. During these months, Jacq met thirty two year old Luke, at her SAE College, and they started going out. Ben had strenuously objected, and fought with his sister. A few months later, eighteen year old Jacq, moved out with Luke, into an Innaloo unit. It was to Luke, Jacq gave credit, for helping her get clean, from her addiction, (when she was homeless and abandoned?).

The next step in Dale's Divorce plan, was to ask to be released, from our marriage vows, to marry Collette. It was at Bibra Lake, a sentimental place, to soften the blow. He slyly suggested an affair with Harold. When I fell apart, sobbing, to the ground, Dale said, "Maybe later". Dale had a divorce agenda, for which he had already hand-picked a psychiatrist, who excluded me as a non-entity, incompatible partner, in a 'Bad marriage', ready for that "Maybe Later". The reconciliation had only ever been a ploy to bide his time and double-dip in a second settlement. Crys did a private official reconciliation ceremony, also at Bibra Lake. After the reconciliation, Dale elected to stay in his Victoria Park flat (no change). At no point did I "Test" the reconciliation, advised in the very book Dale had sent me (Melbourne). Dale introduced me to his new group and Don Laine (my Eagle).

The pub scene, where Jacq and Luke mixed music for their band, was not the best of places to work, especially as they used up all their pays, on drink 'tabs'. Turkey parents, supplied food, when they had nothing in the fridge. Looking back, instead of a rescue, being responsible to them, to tell them to get proper jobs, would have been more appropriate. I had just perpetuated, what Lavender had done with Christine, Will and Beth. When Jacq and Luke broke up, Jacq got a week-end job (still with Luke), at a night club. Jacq stayed friends with all her boyfriends till she was only allowed to keep Luke, because he saved her life (when her mother abandoned her – the lie made up for this purpose). Luke was to become a third partner in her marriage.

Then the biggest mistake of all! To give a loan, that Jacq had begged for, when no bank would lend. And, without contract or the ability of regular jobs, to pay it back. It was for a Music Business (with Luke), but, without any investment from Luke. In hindsight, if a bank wouldn't lend, neither should I have. She returned $150 of the $53,000 and turned the loan, into an unwanted gift, forced down her throat (see Receipts for $150 for loan: Exhibit One, and Thank You card: Exhibit Two) after thanking me 'soooo much' for it. Jacq refused to recant her lies, despite the evidence.

Although Jacq admitted forgetting some things, because of her drug use, she asked me, if I had 'Dementia' and forgotten the gift, made into a loan. Joan once used 'Nanaesk' for the same purpose. When I emailed the evidence, as requested, Joan said she might have a different opinion. Emotionally damaged, Joan's harsh judgement, apparently reflected her, "Difference of opinion" and "Disbelief", of the evidence sent (includes all four 'Exhibits' in this edition), according to Rev. De Visser. Joan wasn't interested in anything I had to say, either. Jacq took her big twin's advice, to get a real job, passed her University Entrance Exam and applied to do Primary School Teaching. Like Joan and Ben, Jacq was an academic after all. I learned to have contracts, for any 'Hand-Up's', and made sure they had good jobs, to make the repayments. As a general rule, family only pay back the principal, no interest.

Beth was in third term, when she met Tom Crooze, at a "Gathering" at Tom's friend, Ned Kelly's place, in Applecross. Had I known, there were drugs (mainly pot), Beth wouldn't have been given a ride there. Tom came to stay for a month. After a month, I asked Tom to leave, as he was a distraction to Beth, and she started to miss school. Beth chose to leave with Tom. Turkeys took responsibility for Beth and Tom, and rented a flat in Hilton. Tom was given a safe, for Beth's ADHD medication. Beth relapsed with an overdose (the first of many to come), when Tom let her have all her medications. In full blown psychosis, she was admitted involuntarily (also the first of many to come), to Alma Street, F.H. Tom should have carried his own knapsack/ responsibility (*Boundaries*) at twenty, and Beth should have stayed home (at seventeen).

Although I had nursing jobs, I did not want another burn out, so financial advise was sought. All three properties, were put on the market. The two Shelley units, with a good deposit included, were first offered to Joan and Ben. They refused, and I suspect they had been advised by Dale, not to get involved with my "Hair-brained Schemes". Ben had once called me a, "Hair-Brained Schemer". Possibly the same reason, why Joan had refused to rent my unit, offered to her, before Crys. Joan and Ben preferred instead, to rent in Maylands, from strangers. Dale and I didn't visit Joan as she was on a time-out from parents, but, Dale and I visited Ben once. After all three properties were sold, a three by one home was purchased in Haynes Court, Kardinya.

A year later, as a reconciled wife, I felt like a week-end prostitute. Jacq once said, this should not be a problem, as we were separated. She had met Collette. Joan, Ben and Jacq, never accepted, the reconciliation (Inscription in gift in Evidence: Exhibit Three).

They accepted Dale's version, that he had only come back to help with Beth (discharged from Alma Street). Pressed by the group, Dale returned to Kardinya, under duress. Apparently, Iris was still sharing intimacies, when she said, "Dale had come back too soon". After returning to Kardinya, Dale sold his Victoria Park flat, and paid off my loan from Bert. Instead of thanking me/us, Bert asked for interest, not paid by family (related to the secret lie). As a thank you, to Dale, I put Kardinya in both names, for 'love and affection'. Beth warned me, not to. She was right, when he stayed the stipulated eighteen months, to get half, in a second settlement.

Dale asked me to get counseling, for awareness of the issues (in his mind, to divorce, not reconcile). The counselor was impressed, at how I had handled the situation, saying she had learned more from me (not unlike A.R.A.F.A.M.I). She told me what I already knew, that Dale blamed me for everything, his illness included (Dr. Peck's Blaming Games). I was the problem he wanted to divorce. Ben once called me the 'Family Problem' he had runaway to the U.K. from. Dale also saw the end of all my savings (for the first time, since 'Retail Therapy'), some to a South African couple, who attended the 'Marriage Enrichment Seminar' with us. Dale told them to keep it (behind my back).

Dale and I had become good friends, with Don. Don diligently kept in touch, with every member of the group. Then when Don rang, Dale took to handing the phone to me, for a woman's opinion. At the same time, Dale suddenly seemed to lose interest, and slept through Group get-together's. At Kardinya, he moved into a single bedroom. He was to go to NZ with me, to see our friend Crys. At the last moment, he changed his mind, and went for a holiday, with his mum and aunts instead. It was around this time, Dale verbalised his tolerance, not love, for a light brown woman. Then Dale started early morning walks with Iris, who lived down the road, at the 'Samson Retirement Village'. He refused to be my, "Coffee Servant". In hindsight, I believe this was a ploy, to get me to leave, as Lewis had tried with Iris, and succeeded. Dale was like his dad – the very thing he had feared the most, at his first Heathcote admission.

I was home on workers comp, with a back injury, which proved too much, for Dale to handle. Dale left, after Don's fifty first birthday party, at the food hall, in Victoria Park, with his boys, then thirteen and fourteen. Gale was seated near both boys, in an attempt to take over from "Dale's poisonous wife" (the only poison was my perfume) for a 'woman's opinion'. I am almost certain, Iris and Gale were privy, to Dale's plans. Dale left for the last time, on 31 July, 2004 after giving me a letter (see date on page of letter in Evidence: Exhibit Four). That "Maybe Later" had come. The letter did ask me to, "Get healthy like an Eagle and find another Eagle, without mental illness" (the theme of all three books).

Bob Hope was the best-man again, of a divorce this time (not marriage), as he drove a removal-van, to pick up Dale's things. While Dale and Bob had a cup of tea, I asked Dale not to do this. Dale replied not to go there. When I went to hug him goodbye, Dale danced out of my reach, and both men laughed, cruelly. I watched a turkey, drive out of my life for good, and an Eagle was born and didn't beg. Beth and Tom, came back to Kardinya, soon after. A week after Dale left, Don proposed to me by phone. "I might ask you to marry me", Don tested, to which I replied, "I might say yes". Joan asked, why I had to remarry, I now believe, the family had had a plan, which did not include a remarriage. In moving on, I had also changed both "Mother's of Origin's" history. Don became a threat, when Dale (who had a key) saw him, pick me up for a date, and I told Dale, we were dating.

First, Dale stalked me at Don's home, at Kennerly Street, Cloverdale. Then came to Cloverdale, with his best mate Bob Hope, to threaten me with court action, if there wasn't a third settlement, for half my super, and supposed millions, in workers comp. They scuttled off like two rabbits, when Don defended me, and swore at them. An appointment with Relationships Australia was next. The lady first asked, who Don was. As soon as I said, "Finance", she quietly gave me back the forms. In reflection, I believe, Dale would have broken up, and reconciled, till there was nothing left. Dale once said, it was only due to my loyalty, faithfulness and long suffering, the marriage had lasted as long as it had. It had been one-sided. An Eagle had stopped "Flapping/Clapping" with a Turkey. Then Dale took to writing letters. The bag of letters, was eventually discarded, by the new owners, of Kennerly Street.

The only thing, holding a Turkey and Eagle together, was the Kardinya property. A letter of consent, was procured, from Dale's Dr. Rude, to attest to his stable mind, to sign an authority, to sell. When the 50:50 settlement was put through, Dale demanded, I give my half to the children, as deposits for their first homes. There's little doubt, the plan included, caring for Bert and Lavender. I refused, and hung up on his rant. The past, no longer, directed my present or future, as Dr. Phil McGraw often says. Dale's Divorce Application, was good to go, after the joint property was settled. When Dale couldn't get his way, with a new application, he hid in Graylands Hospital. Hence, Iris and his doctor's were served on his behalf, by my lawyer. Dale finally got the divorce he asked for. When things didn't go his way, Dale lied in revenge.

> "Liz left me, ran off with my best mate,
> broke up the family, when I was unwell.
> Sold the house from under my feet,
> and took all the Meade money.
> Liz is a liar, don't listen to her."
> The other parents added "Abandonment".

Although there wasn't a "Mummy's Boy", there was a "Daddy's man" (so much for Ben being his own man), and "Daddy's Women and girl" (stuck at thirteen), who went along or stood on Dale's lies. Beth went along, despite knowing the truth/facts (for money, for drugs), more important than standing by her mother. Besides, Joan and Jacq dismissed Beth's witness. Ironically, the first property settlement, to protect assets 'from mental illness', cost me half my house in the second settlement, 'to mental illness'

(Dale's). With his half settlement, Dale purchased a Bentley Duplex.

Dale lost his unit, in a court case, when he took revenge on Dr. Rani, six months later. Thinking he was rid of the 'Family problem', Dale had asked Dr. Rani, to recant her original diagnosis and 'Form Eleven' admission. When she refused, Dale set fire to her practice door. Dr. Rani's insurance company, went after Dale for costs. Dale was de-registered, by the Medical Board, for arson, and charged with perjury, for claiming his wife, had run off and he had had a break down, when a copy of his last letter (Exhibit Four), given to Dr. Rani (as a thank you for her help) showed otherwise.

Looking back, this divorce, had been a long time coming. From an amber light warning, to offering a divorce, when first diagnosed, to a serious suicide attempt, to release me, when I had refused the divorce, to asking for a divorce, at our first separation, and a divorce application (with a book on *Rebuilding When Your Marriage Ends*) sent to my Melbourne workplace. Then asking me, to release him, from our marriage vows, to marry Collette, on my return from Melbourne, and finally in his last letter, "...to find another Eagle, without a mental illness." (Exhibit Four). He walked out on the reconciliation, and followed through on his, "Maybe later" (whispered under his breath). Bert believed Dale and disinherited his daughter and Lavender liked Dale better than Don.

My settlement, went half share, in a home, with Don, at Somers Street, Belmont. Don paid for Beth to fly to Pt. Hedland (and aunt Christine), to mend her broken heart, when she broke up with Tom. Dale gave her $5 at the airport, beating his chest, as a dad. She had also aborted their baby, as there was no future with Tom. When Christine refused to help Beth, it was Don, who drove for two days, to set her up, in her own flat, with a girlfriend named Vanessa. They left all the furniture, we had purchased, and moved to share a house, with another girl. Don paid to transport a car for Beth, so she wouldn't have to walk to work, in the hot Hedland sun. Beth worked as a P/T Pharmacy Assistant and at the local Club.

When the 'godfather' paid for Beth, and her car to return, for university studies, we helped her move, into the student quarters, at Murdoch University. Beth got a P/T job at the South Street Fremantle Pharmacy. The car was never transferred, and Beth let anyone and everyone, drive it. Her multiple DUI's, was paid by the godfather. Beth never paid off Tom's phone bill, and Tom still owes me, for his driving fines. Beth intended to do Pharmacy, or be a Forensic Scientist, like Dale's second girlfriend, Samantha (Sam). Beth was kicked out of Murdoch University, student block, for a DD. She moved into, a shared private house, at Murdoch, with other students. Eagles refused to rescue Beth, but, the godfather did, although he refused to let her stay with him as his Carer.

When Beth burnt the kitchen, while cooking, the house was sold, and she moved in, with Ned and the Kelly family. The entire Kelly family, gave Beth large hand-outs, despite my repeated requests, to charge board. Then Beth was admitted, on our HBF, for stomach pains, at S.J.O.G Hospital, Murdoch, where Bert visited (thanks to Christine telling him, when asked not to), to claim Beth as his own, as he assured her, not to worry, because he had everything for her. Given too much, Beth gave up her job and became wasteful, spoilt and a dependent cripple adult (also from Dr. Phil).

A 'Butterfly', who morphed into a Turkey, with another Turkey (in a threesome with his mother), had circled the 'Mountain of Doom', for twenty seven years. Simultaneously, ending was a thirty year, nursing career and an 'Imitation, Novel, Love, Story'. One Turkey had "...done the best he knew how." (letter in Exhibit Four). Dale still circled Mt. Doom with his 'Three girls'. The other Turkey, chose to become an Eagle, and flew off the mountain, soaring high and strong, with healing in her wings, and found another Eagle, to travel the Highway (of life and for life). Two 'Fruit loops' couldn't live together after all. So, as Turkeys ended, the Eagles began.

CHAPTER NINE

Weddings, Marriages, Funerals, Deaths And Births

This chapter now includes all special occasions, since the first book was published, twelve years ago. It includes weddings attended, marriages and remarriages. All deaths are recorded (one suicide and one unexpected death included). Only some funerals were attended. The births of nine grandchildren (of both Eagles), are recorded. After the Divorce Decree, the Eagles were formally married, at Ascot Gardens, in a simple civil ceremony, witnessed by Joan, her new boyfriend John Farnham, Ben, with new girl friend Tess, Jacq & Beth. Don's sons, Matthew (Matt) and Mark, from his first marriage, were sent an invitation. They were not allowed to attend, by their mum (Don's ex-wife of seven years). Our wedding was followed by a Nando's chicken lunch, at our first home, at Somers Street, Belmont. With Don was fulfilled, that old Secunderabad, prophecy, of 'heart over looks'. Ben said, "It wasn't what I had done, but how" (as Daddy's man).

Jacq and Beth signed as witnesses to our marriage. Our last overseas trip, was a honeymoon to NZ. It was while in NZ, that Crys showed no interest in either of us. She had obviously heard from Dale. I had gone, from a special little sister she never had, to an ex-landlady, ending as 'two ships that passed in the night'. All photographs taken with Crys, were sent to her son. They were no longer friendship memories. After Joan and Ryan broke up, Joan used the wedding money, Dale and I had given her, for a wedding present, to buy some formal clothes, in favour of her shabby single suit, she had worn to court, with multiple coloured shirts, during her 'Article Clerk' days. John Farnham was her new Beau; a police officer, she had met, while having drinks with her colleagues, near the courthouse. It was love and marriage at first sight.

Don and I first met John's parents; Susan & Allan Farnham, over a 'Devonshire Tea' at their place in Duncraig. "You look like Joan", Allan complimented, only to be corrected by Sue, "You mean Joan looks like her mother." We warmed to the Farnham family and their middle son (of three). Dale met John's parents soon after us. Then, via frequent visits, Dale told them (as he had already told everyone else), his version of the separation and divorce, that had supposedly left him destitute, and unable to contribute towards the wedding. Not a word about his lost Bentley unit in the Court Case with Dr. Rani. The Eagles never washed their dirty linen, of the Divorce and remarriage, in public. Not one person checked Dale's one-sided accusations. Pastor Dusty said he had heard (from Dale, no doubt), that I had found myself, "...another fella."

The engagement party, was held by Allan and Sue. The "Mummy's boy" stood with his mother and "first wife", at the front door, to greet the guests. Don and I bypassed the door, and went through the side gate, directly to the party in the backyard. Joan did tell her dad to behave, now that I was remarried, and told us off for not mingling. We sat with strangers, away from Bert (with the Meade's). There was an awkward moment with Thomasina; nothing remarkable. However, sinister not awkward, was when Dale stood at the sweets table, with a butchers knife in his hand. I turned about face, when I saw him, but not before I saw an evil smirk, cross his face. Don did the same and both Eagles believed, Dale intended foul play.

When the sisters had fought over the large sum of money, Jacq got for her music business, to get her big sister off her back, she again used the lie, of her music business loan, turned gift, forced down her throat. Joan felt 'Entitled' (a stronghold in the sequel) to the same 'Gift' for her wedding. No doubt Dale had also instructed, to get as much of the 'Taken' Meade money (before I gave it to Don and his sons), as I had not listened, to give them deposits for their homes. I now believe this was the reason Joan asked me along (not as a mum), to shop for her wedding dress, with Sue and best friend Shirley. Many happy hours arm in arm had followed, with Joan picking a beautiful dress and veil (which Don paid for). Joan asked me to organise the venues (and pay for it is now presumed), but, I gave her the quotes. A 'Breakfast invite' to their Sorrento home, didn't net them $53,000 (Jacq's loan) for John's new boat (they had hinted at), to replace the one he sold, to pay for their wedding.

Rev. A. De Visser's First Draft on *Healing For Damaged Emotions*, also pointed out that emotional damage can, "... manifest as a judgemental spirit...", and judge the eagles, Joan most definitely did. The anger, followed by rage and bitterness, came later (also strongholds in the Sequel). Eagles were unaware of either the expectation, judgement or anger. Besides, Joan as a lawyer, would have known, that divorce settlements were split equally between Husband and wife, and not given by one party to their adult children. Of such is Emotional Damage. De Visser also claimed, "Hurting people hurt people". Punishment followed, for not coming to the party, or wedding, as the case was.

It began with the, "Bridal Breakfast" in Ocean Reef Coffee House, a few days later. I was relegated to the end of the long table, opposite a very cold Sue Farnham, who pointedly turned towards her friend, seated next to her (body language spoke volumes) and ignored me for the entire breakfast. Shirley & Mrs Watsonia occupied the seats of honour, next to the bride-to-be. "Accumulated hurts can come out, as uncontrollable fits of anger" according to Rev. De Visser, and they certainly did, in Joan's explosive anger, when I was short just $2 for Beth's breakfast. Joan asked me to stop, "Trying to be the mother". It was Joan, who was trying to be the mother of her siblings, and mother of her mother.

The wedding was held at the Kings Park Gardens. I rode in the limousine, with the bride and bridesmaids; Jacq and Beth, Shirley (married) was Matron of Honour and seated next to Joan (again, not the mother of the bride). I was literally a distant mum. Shirley gave me her camera, to give to her mum, interrupting my musings, on what a lovely bride, my eldest daughter made. In giving me the camera, it was supposed to have deterred me, from trying to walk Joan down the aisle (I learned later), although I had done, precisely what I was instructed. Two 'Fruit Loops' were not permitted to 'Give the Bride away'. Joan opted to walk herself down the aisle, with John meeting her half-way. Then both walked together to where Pastor Dusty waited.

Next punishment was the frosty reception from the newly weds, when I welcomed John into the family. As I arrived, I got a cold peck on the cheek from Ben (as the 'Family Problem' not mum). The Meade family were not invited although Gale, Max and Thomasina showed up at the nuptials. Lavender hugged and kissed me, as she congratulated me, on the marriage of my eldest, dressed in a shabby old dress, she had hand-sewn, and an old sweater, beside a smartly suited Bert. It was to be, the last time, I saw my mother alive. I now treasure this memory, as I sadly regret, wiping her kiss away, and not paying her more attention, or simply making sure, she had a nice outfit, for her first and only grandchild's wedding. But, Bert and Lavender had actually been uninvited to the wedding, some six months earlier, by Joan.

Joan had brought her grandfather to our place in Belmont, to re-open the 2003 Guardianship (by Dale and myself) as Bert had had a change of heart. But when Bert learned a Public Trustee was to handle Lavender's 50% of all financial affairs, and he would lose control of the savings, Bert scared Lavender into believing I was trying to put her away in a nursing home (again). She went with Bert to get their lawyer to cancel it, making Joan very angry. When the person (supposedly) with all Meade funds, didn't come through, with paying for the wedding, and Bert offered a $20,000 (I had unknowingly, happily approved) wedding gift, the godfather was re-invited to Joan's wedding. The first we knew, was when we saw my parents, at the nuptials, and later at the reception.

The reception and dinner were no warmer. Sue and Allen ignored us, while my parents sat, with Iris and Dale, at the farthest corner of the room. I was to take care of the flowers for the venue, and got the most wilted bunch, as a thank you, after Sue Farnham, Mrs. Watsonia and Shirley. Then the clincher, after thanking his parents, for all their help with the wedding, John said that I was more excited than the bride and groom, without so much as a mention, of Joan's wedding dress gift (soon after a divorce and Dale had contributed nothing). We spoke to a friend of the bride all evening. I did a little dancing, but, always distanced from Joan, Ben, Jacq and Beth.

It did not improve the next day, at the opening of wedding gifts, at Sue & Allan Farnham's place. Our wedding card with $100 must have been the last straw. Meantime, the abuse of my mother by Bert continued. She was excluded from Bert's Health insurance, phone, and food (kept in a locked spare bedroom), because she had refused, to contribute to the household. Her self-neglect worsened, when instead of buying and taking her (newly diagnosed) Diabetic medication (or forgot it in her Dementia), she remembered to give all her pension away (the only control she had had) to Christine, Will and Beth. Her food was fried bread crumbs, with borrowed money, from Dr. Rani's cleaner, and Jam sachets from her church.

It was already too late, when the starvation, had reduced the once beautiful woman, to a skeleton. Last minute, Bert guiltily tried to force-feed Lavender her medications. Without a health fund, she was admitted again, as a public patient, at Fremantle Hospital (as it would've cost Bert $800/day at S.J.O.G. Murdoch). I did visit at the first admission (she probably forgot it, and the purple things I gave her, which Bert took credit for, despite my docket for the purchases). The second admission was portrayed as not serious, and that she "Hated the sight of me", anyway, although Beth said, she was asking to see me. My one solace, was that her youngest sister Jade, did visit (and disliked me even more, for not visiting).

Lavender died, from multi-organ failure (the preventable complications of Diabetes), after being four days in a coma. I hoped she was taken quickly, before nurses heard her starving, stomach, much as I had, when I nursed patients in a coma. My submission to the Tribunal came too late for my mother. It is hoped, it would help others, with abusive carers. Bert literally abused Lavender to death. I got a phone call from a police officer (not John, Bert or Joan) to inform me, of my mother's passing. Joan was too upset at losing "her mother" (based on a father's lie). I know my parents neither fell in love again, nor did Lavender die of a broken heart, because of me (another 'Blame Game').

Eagles were now living in the newly, (owner) built 'granny flat-shed home' (intended for Bert and Lavender), in the large 900m2 backyard, and rented out the old house in front. The rent augmented a disability pension, as a retired nurse. Don gave up, his mechanical business, to care for me, R.T. Kiyosaki's 'Cash Flow' concept, of *Rich Dad, Poor Dad*, in action.

Before Christine could fly down, for our mother's funeral, a meeting was held in a coffee shop, by Joan, for afternoon tea (except Don and I), where the funeral arrangements were made. I was put off till late afternoon, when this meeting finished, before we could call in to pay my respects, to a cold Bert (directly connected to a secret lie). The daughters were delegated the 'Wake' (which Eagles got to pay for). Thankfully, Dale was not invited to the wake. All my children, behaved like they had lost their mother, and ignored me. Don's younger son Mark, was the only one to give me any sympathy for my loss. Ben flew back to Perth, from the U.K. for the funeral, no doubt bankrolled by the godfather. I did get a floppy hug, as I sobbed 'Sorry". In hindsight, a mistake, as parents don't owe children an apology or it would have become a '*Never Ending Story*' (a movie).

Dale, the Watsonia family and Farnham's, were invited to the funeral, to support Joan, as it appeared to be generally accepted, that 'Nana had raised her grandchildren' as 'Photos didn't lie'. Christine had whispered in my ear, that everyone was saying this, to her too, about Will. Uncle Monte's daughter; the only one to invite me and Dale to her wedding, gave me a sympathy wish and chat. This is when Dale made a public announcement of having 'Four Mongrels'. He was quickly shushed by pastor Dusty (asked by Joan, to do the Funeral service).

A week later, via a sms Bert's try-hard daughter, invited all for my mother's plaque, and ashes laying ceremony. This Eagle took her place back, by not attending, done in private, a year later. It was during the two week clean up, that I discovered the B & W family photographs, Lavender had stashed away from Bert (who had thrown all photographs out, to hurt Lavender, not unlike my burnt photo albums by Dale/Bert the second). The purple handbag, was hidden in her closet. It contained letters in my mother's handwriting. All her letters began with, "today he hit me...". It had broken my heart, to see Lavender's half packed suitcase, she had planned to take with her, on her visit to Pt. Hedland, to visit Christine (cruelly cancelled by Christine).

Her bedraggled nurse uniforms and shoes, in the closet, had brought fresh tears, rolling down my cheeks. After the room was cleaned, and her amber collection donated, Bert had dropped a bombshell. He hoped I didn't mind sharing my inheritance, with my four children, in equal shares (because Joan had looked at the Will and deemed Don and his sons, a danger). For this one fifth share, "You Lizzy girl must look after me and Divorce Don, to get your share of inheritance". "I hope you don't mind going to a nursing home", I retorted, hurt and rejected . I pleaded with Bert to reconsider. His Will was iron clad he informed me, with a smirk. This too, was explained by that 'Secret Lie', after his death. Then Bert told us to leave, as Joan and John were coming over. I had asked Bert why we had to leave. I found out a year later.

Joan had sent an sms, to let us know, Bert was in hospital, which was my job as NOK. When I asked her (by sms reply) if she was telling us as Bert's NOK, Joan asked how we knew. Joan and John had turned up at our place the same evening, because of sending Joan "Abusive sms's". Joan had intimidated, standing over me as a lawyer (for heavens sake) not my daughter. In punishment, Joan had banged her mobile phone, on our kitchen table, and threatened we would neither see her nor her children ever again. Then John had asked Bert's daughter, "Who else was there?" 'John's quizzical look when I replied, "What am I?", has stayed with me, ever since. John simply didn't know what he didn't know (Dr. Phil McGraw). The answer lay, in that secret lie. Bert's obsolete old Will was returned. It had been employed, with trickery (based on lies), to let an Eagle act as NOK, but, under Joan's authority.

The next wedding was Jacq's and JK's, the following November (like Joan's), who were now in a close-by unit in Rivervale. The first we knew of this wedding, was when we called into the butchers shop, at the Belmont Forum Shopping Centre, to say hello to Jacq. It was not Jacq, but, another girl who she worked with, who told us that Jacq boasted a new engagement ring, which she then reluctantly showed us. Had we not seen the ring, Eagles believe, an invitation, would not have been forthcoming. The engagement party, was at the Willeton pub, where Jacq and JK first met. JK like John Farnham, is in the middle of three sons, of Susan and Peter Kennedy. They were in Adelaide, and to come for the wedding, and stayed with JK and Jacq in Rivervale.

There was to be no formal meet and greet with the senior Kennedy parents, as there was, "...not enough food to go around, and Peter ate too much". Jacq didn't want any money for her wedding, because, I always "...asked back for any money given". Dale's last letter (Exhibit Four) had referred to the money, and said to, "Tell Jacq & Joan it was me claiming the money to be paid back. It was. When I get manic, I like to settle old scores. I don't know my boundaries." Even Dale at some level, knew it was a loan. After a 'Family Meeting' at their place (not a meal invite), JK dubbed us as a, "Tolerated Nonsense at Special Occasions". Luke or, "Butt-head, big brother", was to be her, "brides-mate", till I strenuously objected.

Most unlike Joan's wedding, Jacq had chosen a simple tarp, erected at the riverside in Bicton. The 'Other Mother' (since the age of seven) was M.C. and at the unit when Don dropped me off. I got the cold shoulder, from Jacq's sister-in-law, who was doing Jacqs hair. Mother Joan had competed with me in the hallway, to get to the Bride first and help her with her outfit. I got to Jacq first. Jacq always believed she was the ugly duckling. In her wedding outfit, taller than both her sisters, she looked to me, to be the most beautiful, and very much a, "Meade". This time there was no Limo-ride and Eagles went straight to the venue, where pastor Dusty waited. Jacq also walked herself down the aisle. Ben greeted the 'Family problem', with a pat on the back. Dale and Sam, brought Bert, to Jacq's wedding. Godfather paid for the wedding, and 'Father figure, ex-boyfriend' Luke, gave a big money gift, on their money tree. We gave the usual $100 from a 'Tolerated Nonsense At Special Occasions'.

After the ceremony, Iris, Bert, the bride, Joan, and Beth spoke exclusively, to Dale and Sam, who sat isolated, under a tree, near the riverbank, kissing and cuddling. The Forensic Scientist, did ask Beth how I had put up with Dale. After the fiasco, at Joan's wedding dinner, Eagles refused JK's last minute invitation, to a dinner, after the wedding. A 'Father-Figure', (not family) gave the speech for the bride. When JK thanked the 'special egg and sperm donor' for making a special Jacq, the reason for both wedding invitations, became apparent, especially after, spotting the satisfied smirk on Joan's face. Designed to publicly insult, humiliate and punish parents, underpinned by the disrespect taught by 'The Other Parents' and Dale. Joan once told me, every time I had chastised her or her siblings, Dale had rolled his eyes behind my back. Dale's lies to discredit both Eagles, cemented the disrespect. The Bride told Don, "Not a word out of you!" Ben drunk had walked away and tipsy Beth came home with us.

In June, Jacq announced her pregnancy. Eagles were relegated to the, "Friends" Baby shower (not with family). Eagles gave the baby gift to best friend Candy, who answered the door, making an excuse of another engagement. JK sent an sms to announce the birth of their son (now thirteen). With red hair and blue eyes he was a Kennedy. "Mother" Joan was first to visit and no doubt Bert, Dale and Sam (on FB with baby afterwards). Then came the restricted, visitation hours, for the 'Tolerated egg donor at special occasions' and 'That man' (a wife stealer and brainwasher). First, it was on the weekend, then it was between one and three, during week days. Eagles didn't go on any days, because Jacq still refused to refute her lies. JK like John, simply didn't know what he didn't know (Dr. Phil). Besides, they had believed their wives and father-in-law, their word against a discredited mother.

Beth was first diagnosed, in 2008. Beth has two alter egos, although lacks insight into both (Bipolar part). One is an abused seven year old, the other a traumatised teen. Stuck at thirteen, this childish ego, wants to be looked after, (instead of looking after her son) and is terrified of being alone. This alter-ego sabotages independent living, aided and abetted, by an adult, "dependent cripple" (Dr. Phil McGraw) created by Hand-outs. Beth is aware at some level, sharing both traumas with all her friends, but, denied them when confronted. Beth has no money management skills and either is homeless, or lives with anyone as long as she wasn't alone. It is hoped, Beth will listen and seek Therapy and Rehab., rather than steal (for drugs) or self-destruct (self-harm or overdose).

After Dale and Sam had broken up, I got the news (in hospital at the time), that Dale had jumped off, a building in Fremantle (Beth has threatened to jump off a bridge). As for Dale's apparent, "Suicide", at fifty five, it was first coined an 'Accidental Suicide' in the sequel. The seventeen year old, reckless teen, finally succeeded, just as that ED doctor predicted. Dale had Schizo-affective Disorder, as well as Bipolar II Disorder. After Lewis passed away, Dale had had a meeting, with his siblings, at

Bibra Lake. They decided, their dad had Schizophrenia. So the 'Personality Disorder' had also been Schizo-Affective Disorder. There is a distinct possibility, that Dale's maternal grandmother, who committed suicide, when Iris was sixteen, was also Schizo-Affective Disordered. Dale had had no insight into his own persona's (the Bipolar part). Had it been known, divorce (with sole custody) was the only option.

Beth ended with another DD charge after Dale's death. Mother Joan rescued Beth and slapped Beth (mother-like). To rescue is being, "Responsible for", instead of "Responsible to" Beth, to carry her own knapsack/consequences, for her actions", as Cloud and Townsend advocated, in their book on *Boundaries.* Contrary to what an Eagle mother would've done, the rescue by the lawyer (Joan) and Police Officer (John), stopped Beth learning from her mistakes, and/or consequences of her actions.

After Dale's death, one final call was made to Bert, to request him to re-install me, as his daughter and NOK. Bert claimed he had lost like a son, and hung up. Our absence at Dale's funeral was apparently 'noticed', according to Beth. Iris had been a, 'Pillar of Strength' at her son's funeral (for Joan). Pastor Dusty did the funeral service. Then, Beth announced the suicide had been added to the blame list. There would've been little doubt, both 'Blame Scapegoats' would've been unceremoniously escorted out, in the ultimate public humiliation, in the presence of all family, and professionals, at the funeral. Eagles in the 'Power of three' (in the sequel), were not powerful enough to cause the actions of others (Dr. Phil McGraw). Apart from getting into the thought processes, where the actions began (also discussed in the sequel), no one can make someone kill themselves.

Meantime, Matt met Esther, married and had two sons, eleven months apart. Neither John nor Joan informed us of the birth of their first baby boy, born same year. The boys are now in high school and final year primary school.

The unexpected death, was fifty two year old Christine, after an operation to unblock both her neck (Carotid) arteries. This operation had a small mortality risk from stroke. Sadly, Christine was that statistic. After a phone call chat, to reassure her, I never would've guessed, it was for the last time. A Coroners Report into her death, released three years later, to Channel Nine News, reported on, "Warning signs missed in WA hospital death." Further, "Medical staff didn't identify or notice, possible developing complications, or the warning signs following, 'uncomplicated technically successful' surgery". She had, "died from a catastrophic stroke, the day after she was sent home from hospital" (thanks to the bed-shortage in the Public Sector and high blood pressure, not brought under proper control, before discharge). Another unexpected death, was the middle child, of Max and Thomasina. The 'Middle child club' had lost one of their own.

Eagles were invited to the funeral, and wake (as family), by second husband Brett. Seated in front, was the godparent-godfather with **his** children. Beth and Ned, now an 'Item', were seated on the opposite side. Ben and English nurse and fiance' Alice, sat at the end of the row (presume to beat a hasty exit, should the family problem approach). Wearing dark glasses, an Eagle was thankful to sneak a peek, at her adult offspring, all be it, their backs. Bert had shown no interest in his only remaining kin (also relative to that secret lie). The request to sit next to Bert, made by John without greeting or condolence, was declined. Joan had made several attempts, to bring the designated Nurse-carer to heel, even to the use of photos, of her children, as a grandmother-bribe. But the Eagle remained resolute, for eleven years.

The first book, along with family heirlooms, and a card, (to thank the 'run-away-silent-son', for not inviting the family problem, to play pretend happy families, at his wedding) was sent to Burns Beach, where the engaged couple stayed (with John and Joan). When Ben couldn't find room, in his suitcase for the book, it was skim-read by Joan. Joan's only comment, was that it was, "...mostly accurate". Ben was married in the U.K. the following year. The wedding was attended by the 'Other Mother' with her baby daughter and aunt Gale. The aunt that once couldn't recall Joan's name, when she had given Joan a rare birthday present, was now a close confidante. Ben and Alice, divorced a year later, without any children. Years and many failed relationships later, Ben was to finally settle at forty one, with his first child (English grandchild returns to 12% English Roots).

Joan and Jacq had had daughters two months apart, the same year. Jacq's son is in second year high, and both granddaughters are in year five. None of them have met their only, remaining, maternal, grandparent. They had a, "big grandpa" (Great grandfather Bert) and big grandma (great grandmother Iris), as well as one set of paternal grandparents.

According to best friend June on FB, Bert had made a last trip to Podanur to grieve his daughters loss. He had tried to get June's mother (then eighty four) to look after him, as he no longer had a house to return to, thanks to the consequence of, Bert's iron-clad Will. June's mum refused. Bert stayed at the granny flat, built in Joan's home, till he was put in a 'Nursing Home' (as warned), with Dementia (to discredit any Will changes after Urbahns Crescent was sold and distributed). Joan had exhausted every effort, to get a 'try-hard mother' to take on 'The Burden', even Relationships Australia, and offering to be NOK for the Eagles. When an Eagle stood her ground, punishment followed. The Eagle was excluded from Bert's Nursing Home, and they wouldn't give out any information.

After being sent back from Me-n-u, Beth and Ned neither married nor bought a house, but, got pregnant, while Beth lived with Ned, at his dad's second investment property. It was also against her own better judgement (Beth had not wanted to put, any child, through what she had endured, since the age of one). Beth's baby, boy had been conceived in desperation (homelessness). For Beth, having a baby, was about money (Ned's $700 a week allowance, prostitute-like, for drugs). When pregnant Beth was refused, to have her baby at Me-n-u, Eagles were uninvited to the birth, in favour of 'Mother' Joan, who looked after her, during her pregnancy. We found out about the birth of her boy, not from Beth or Ned, but, posted on FB by a, 'friend' of the family. Big Nana Iris didn't make it to see this great grandson. She suffered a stroke and died before the birth.

Three years later, Joan permitted Beth to inform us of Bert's stroke, and the name of the Nursing home. Beth got a visit in hospital, at the same time, when Eagles met Beth's little two year old, blue eyed, blonde son. After a call to the nursing home, to speak to Bert, the visit only served, for closure for the Eagle. Bert was informed, of the facts, surrounding the departure of Dale, his divorce to marry Collette and the re-marriage. It had elicited a wide-eyed Bert, who could do little but grunt in response. He was a shadow of a man, without his trademark moustache. It was a loving goodbye, even though Bert never opened his eyes, or reached out with his good arm. It is hoped he didn't die angry, but, did die forgiven. Eagles did not attend the funeral, and a 'Tribute to a Dad' was not read out; the final punishment.

A picture of Bert at the late Christine's remarriage, and indifference in comparison, to the Eagle's remarriage, spelled out the 'Secret Lie', Lavender, Bert and Christine had taken to their graves. The lie, that Lavender had used, to convince Bert, to give Tarrant Way, Bateman, to Christine, and stop that DNA test he had wanted, spelled, *I was the Illegitimate one*. This explained the rejection since then. As the Ancestry DNA would attest, Bert had disowned his very own "Lizzy girl". As such, Bert was my 'Burden' not Joan's (as she often said). Thus I was obliged to him, for having been raised as his own, and only deserved one fifth of the inheritance (without a life of my own). I was not family, therefore had to pay interest on a loan.

It was Bert who hated the sight of me, not Lavender. Lost was eleven years without a dad and twenty eight of rejection. In the end, he couldn't even bear to look at me or touch me. Angry or forgiven, Bert died without ever knowing my Dewar, Ancestry DNA. I am the last of his line. Sadly, Bert had even preferred Dale like a son, over an illegitimate daughter, and did not care when a son-in-law (Patrick) had stolen from her. This finally explained the look of consternation, on John Farnham's face, when I had asked him 'What I was', after a discussion of why Joan was NOK, in my stead, and he had asked, "Who else was there?" I am certain, John believed me illegitimate, but, was sworn to secrecy, by Bert.

Eagles got to attend Mark's marriage to Martha, in a small (Covid-19 safe) civil ceremony in Perth, with a few friends, and his (half) sister, the only family present. Their daughter, the first Miss Laine, was born a few months later. We are now the proud grandparents of Don's three grandchildren. We hope there will be at least one more playmate, once first time parents, get over a teething baby girl. This little girl, the first Miss Laine, was born just ten days before her grandfather, and will be one this year.

Ironically, Bert had his improved race of great-grandchildren, but, without his name and rejected the one with his name. With the death of Bert, all 'Family of Origin' liars were gone, but, not their legacies of secrets, lies and mental illness. Iris was solely responsible, for her lie of omission. Iris wasn't much of a pillar of strength after all. A rebuilt, strong, positive, mature, Eagle couldn't do much about the past. The damage was done and couldn't be undone. The only thing left to do, was to manage it. Eagles trumped the 'baddest things' of lies, with truth or evidence based facts. The mental illness legacy can only be managed by a Guardian, Public Trustee, and the Mental Health Team, supported by Eagles. To manage both legacies, the Eagle went into 'Damage Control', before 'Letting go'.

CHAPTER TEN

Damage Control And Letting Go...

With both families of origin gone, the People of The Lie, that remained are adult children. "Daddy's man and women" and 'Daddy's girl' (for her own selfish needs) are gone too, with daddy's demise. No matter how much Jacq had wanted it, dead people couldn't wait for an Eagle, to come to her senses (when she never lost them). The weddings and funerals had disrespect written all over it. Disrespect was taught by fathers of lies and the other parents. The public humiliation, and punishment, also had shame attached, for the secret lie. Lies, blame and derogatory, demeaning terms, don't define Eagles. When Joan, Ben, and Jacq, and to a lesser extent Beth, clearly showed, they didn't want their mother or a grandmother in their lives, clearly it was best to step away. Although Joan and Jacq had apologised for being difficult teens, an Eagle mum, let Joan, Ben and Jacq go in 'Just Love' (coined in the sequel), and had Joan, Ben, Jacq and Beth, legally removed from her Will. It is hoped, this edition, with it's limited evidence, will one day be read, by these grandchildren (as adults), who won't otherwise know, what they don't, or know, what their grandma knows/knew, as well as the rich heritage, they inherit.

The last time, Joan made contact, was eleven years ago. Joan is forty four and lives her dream in a mansion, on the beach. Ben did not want to be found on FB, and has been a silent son, in the U.K. for sixteen years. Ben is forty two and remains in the U.K. It has been fourteen years, since Jacq called in, to announce her first pregnancy. Jacq repeatedly refused to recant her lies, or heed the warnings, of having an ex-partner in her marriage. Eagles believe it has ended or will end in Divorce (her FB site is gone). Once trust is gone, no relationships are possible (Dr. Cloud and Dr. Townsend), only forgiveness (*Dead Man Walking* by Sr. H. Prejean), and letting them go to the consequences, in 'Just Love'. Besides, when you, "Choose the action, you also choose the consequences" (Dr. Phil). The visit to Beth's hospital, was three years ago. An Eagle mum re-connected, when Beth called from hospital six years ago. It was mostly as an adviser, daughter-advocate and support of her team (for a mental Health history).

As a lawyer (with her own legal firm), Joan was able to get guardianship over Beth's affairs, six years ago, to manage her share of Bert's inheritance, when Urbahns Crescent was sold. Beth (when unwell) has attempted to remove this Guardian, twice so far, without success. In her lucid moments, which are generally short lived, she concedes this is the best and safest and admits lies told, as well as, needing Rehab. for drug use. The guardian also manages Beth's Disability Support Pension, and gives her a nominal weekly allowance. At thirty eight, she remains dependent on co-patients, friends or anyone, to house and feed her, even drug dealer-boyfriends and drug users. Beth once said, all she needed was to be looked after (like a child), and money (for drugs for the teen addict).

The long term drug use, made Beth a people-user, and a thief. It was the theft of $5000, from her future father-in-law, that cost the marriage and being a part of a stable family. Again Beth was denied learning from the consequences of her theft, when Ned paid his dad back and stopped Beth being charged with Stealing. As she had done at sixteen, Beth tried to get herself diagnosed with ADHD, to get Amphetamines, till the Guardian intervened. Cough mixture Sudafed, was used as a 'Speed' substitute, till these Scripts were also cancelled, by tracking the new G.P. Beth then turned to Meth/ice, as the mentally ill often do, according to her treating psychiatrist. At $100 a hit, her allowance, doesn't stretch to three doses. In her lucid moments, she has wished she never touched the stuff and asked for Rehab. Beth once asked for my savings for a car. With a suspended drivers Licence, this was a ploy, to get her hits, or pay back drug-debts, before they bashed her again. Eagles have repeatedly refused, to look after Beth's inner child, or cater to an addict inner teen (where Beth is stuck). So, home was never an option. Beth is infamous for police escorts/welfare checks, multiple ambulance admissions (over fifty five a year) and stomach pumps, for overdoses and self-harm. Sadly, she is a regular, at both mental health hospitals.

Beth goes to hospital, either via ambulance or voluntarily, to detox, then either self discharges, walks out, after smoking a cigarette, or goes AWOL. Beth is a great pretender and lies through her teeth (as teens do), but, as an adult, knows her rights. If she is well, they cannot chase her, or keep her against her will. Of such are the restrictions on a Mental Health Certificate's (for involuntary admissions) or a CTO (can't find a better word for certified insane). Upon every discharge, Beth returns to her drugs, and repeats the cycle. Beth stays wherever she can use her allowance exclusively for the drugs. However, the elicit drugs, destabilises the mental illness. Homelessness is by choice, as Beth has been unable to stay alone, at any number of places, rented on her behalf, by her Guardian. The last place, was left empty, and used for drug-storage, so it was cancelled. Meantime, her son has just turned six and she is an absent mum.

After Ned and Beth split up, Ned got sole custody. When Ned's parents divorced, the mentally ill grandma moved out, making it more stable. Beth and Ned remained in an on-again, off-again relationship, for a short while. Ned brought their son into hospital, to visit his mother (when stable and off drugs). It was on one of these visits, that we had met the two year old. Ned had appeared nonchalant, and indifferent at our visit. Eagles hazard a guess, manipulative Beth had engineered it. Ned did not make any overtures, and all sms messages went unanswered, even the ones, notifying of Beth's admissions. An Eagle, had the pleasure of giving a 'Tonka Truck' to the only grandchild, she will ever meet. Thanks to Beth, this child's grandfather, will be posted a copy of this book, for his eighteenth birthday. After being a patient advocate, the Eagle became a daughter-advocate, when the team asked her to join as part of the solution.

The Eagle mum, became 'Responsible To' the adult, in 'Just Love', for the teen, in 'Tough Love', and for the child in 'unconditional love', for the best most comprehensive care possible. Regular update emails with the Guardian and both teams, kept everyone abreast, of Beth's whereabouts, phone contact (particularly when she irresponsibly threw her new phone away), and if she was taking her prescribed medications. In an attempt to break the six year cycle, of co-patients, living together, co-dependently (not unlike Fruit loops or Turkeys in a single bedroom unit), the Guardian appointed an accommodation specialist, to work with the mental health teams, to look at appropriate long and short term solutions. The Eagle went to the very top, to establish the criteria required, for the long term solution. Beth has been presented with the short term, for 'Supported living'. The long term for a few years, is for regular 'B.M.T.' (holistic to reconcile the persona's), and Rehab. It is hoped Beth takes up these offers, sooner than later, to be the person she can be, and the mother, her son needs. After doing the best possible, it was time to let Beth (now thirty eight) go, to the consequences of her choices, for her life and that of her son.

Then the Eagles set out to make a difference. There were not going to be any more, "Other parents", "Other Wife", "Stolen Generation" or a, "Stolen Million Dollar Inheritance". Only, "Hand-up's". Both stepsons were given, "Hand-Up's", as they worked, married, bought homes and had families. Eagles, were regarded and honoured, at weddings, and the births of three grandchildren (Don's). Matt and Esther, bought their first home, in Me-n-u, which afforded five years, of babysitting two delightful little boys. Then, to attend the local Primary school, for sports carnivals, classroom activities, as honoured grandparents.

Matt and Esther bought their second home, in the local town, to save Matt commuting, an hour each way, to and from work. Both wives are stay at home mums, and the grandchildren thrive on love and stability. Son's respect their wives, just like Don does. All grandchildren know to love, honour and obey (till eighteen) parents, who are the boss, never grandparents (except when babysitting). Grandparent visitations, are strictly curtailed, by pre-arranged appointments, made with husband and wife, and never, 'drop in'. Most important of all, a "Re-built", Eagles marriage, with the 'Three C's' (commitment, companionship and communication), is the best example, for Matt and Mark, after their own parents had divorced. This is precisely what healthy Families, and Rebuilt Marriages, with 'Healing for damaged emotions', and 'Boundaries', are made of.

As a Butterfly and Turkey, I couldn't have known what I didn't. I finally forgave her, for doing the best she knew how. The Butterfly turned Turkey, had faced and risen to the challenges, as a single, sole, provider, mother, when the late Dale first left, doing what she had to do, to provide for all four teenage children. She got her career (she disliked) back, by going back to university (at forty). She neither turned to drugs nor alcohol, and did not chase other men (to rescue her). Of course she couldn't help but be a, "Not all present or all there mum" as a working single mum. When she failed to get sole custody, she returned to abuse, to protect her offspring, till they were adults, and only then moved on. An Eagle does not owe any apology, to adult children (Rabbi H.S. Kushner).

A phone call, from my long lost nephew Will, pre-empted a long awaited apology, and confession, he had 'stuffed up on elicit drugs'. With his prison record, Will felt hopeless. Will was suicidal and asked "what he should do about it?" The question first posed in my sequel, instead of, "Why me?" Advised not to despair, he chose Centre-Link, to get back his life, after his 'Carer' role for his sick dad ended. Patrick developed Emphysema – the dreaded slow death of smokers disease (reminded me of that first death, experienced as a student nurse). Will has a life after his caring role is over, so while he is a carer, he is doing something about, life after being a 'Carer'.

Thanks to my late sister's FB page, I also have Dewar first cousins, from the U.K. and Eastern States of Australia, back in my life, after over fifty years. These cousins gave loving tributes, to their uncle Bert, and condolences, to his grieving daughter. As for the Brady bunch, I did not miss what I never had. All thirteen Dewars, must be having, a reunion party in Heaven, Dewar cousin Susan (I met at eleven) suggested. Cousin Susan, is also an author-publisher, of three best selling books, on Amazon, as well as a, "Trekking queen". You could call them all, "My distant first cousins". Ex-sister in law Anne's son (also), named Matthew (like my stepson), joined the FB family (as an ex-nephew?).

Thanks to a first cousin brother Steve, also on FB, in the U.K., there is a "Dewar Family Tree". It traced all the way back, to a third time Scottish great grandfather, William Dewar. Although Christine was illegitimate, Will has been added to the Dewar family tree, and on FB as kin, in 'Just love'. Will is aware of Lavender's secret lie. If my truth trickles back to the Podanur gossip-vine, and uncle Grant, it will be a bonus. For all the FB friends who blocked me, for the gossip, your loss! Except for June's family in Podanur, people I don't know, or knew for the last two years before leaving, no longer matter, after nearly half a century, in my adopted country. Eagles are proudly Australian, with rich heritages. When Allan and Sue-Lee Bright visited (a few years after Dale's funeral), to insult the Eagles, all friends of 'The Lie/s', were let go.

It is not exclusive, to one family, but, all families dealing in secrets, lies and mental illness. To marry or not, to have children, how many, or not at all. Some choices were taken away for eagles, like the choice, of who one married. Even so, as already discussed in the sequel, and earlier, every choice begins with a thought, or mindset (attitude). It is up to the individual, to modify their own behaviours, by changing or interrupting their thinking (as postulated in the sequence) or get the help they need to make the right choices. Mindsets, are particularly difficult, for any professional to change. Hence 'Holistic' B.M.T proposed in the sequel, to change mindsets and thoughts, or interrupt negative thought patterns, to change outcomes (based on the premise, that every action began with a thought).

The Eagle made sure, Beth was given the best chance, to choose, Rehab. and Therapy, to unlearn bad habits, stabilise her mental health, so she can be the person, she was born to be, and the mother, she was meant to be. The alternative to overcome, is to succumb, self construction instead of self-destruction (suicide). Like the two poles of the disorder, these are 'Bipolar Extremes' and a kind of 'Bipolar Management', of the bad thing i.e. the inherited mental health legacy. While there's life there's hope. The knowledge of the mental illness, is power with wisdom, to overcome or manage it.

The facts or truth have been presented. So, take a leaf out of this book. Don't be stuck or get stuck, in the past, as an immature 'Butterfly' or a 'Fruit Loop Turkey' on a mountain of doom, circling your life away asking, "Why me?" (in Self-Pity). Become an optimistic, rebuilt, self-assured, healthy, eagle, and rise above all the negative bad things, manage or overcome them, by doing something about it. To learn from mistakes, not repeat them, and only repeat successes, is the key to successful management, and get with the Rebuilt, Pro-Life, Overcoming, Powerful and Optimistic *Eagles On The Highway* (of life, for life).

THE END?
OR
A NEW BEGINNING?

ACKNOWLEDGEMENTS

Thank you to the Heads of the Mental Health Department, Mental Health Teams at Fiona Stanley Hospital and Fremantle Hospital, and Office of the Public Advocate, for your diligent, dedicated and unwavering support.

REFERENCES

Cloud and Townsend, Doctors, *Boundaries*, U.S.A. Zondervan Publishing House, 2001.

De Visser, A., Rev., *Healing For Damaged Emotions*, First Draft, Sri Lanka, Kithu Sevan Study Series, 2000.

Fisher, B., *Rebuilding When Your Relationship Ends*, Australia, Footprint Books, 2001.

Kiyosaki, R.T., *Rich Dad, Poor Dad*, Australia, 1998.

Kushner, H.S., *When Bad Things Happen To Good People*, U.K., Pans Book Ltd., 1981.

Laine, D. Elizabeth, *Eagles On The Highway*, Australia Inspiring Publishers, 2014.

McGraw, Phil, Dr. *The Dr. Phil Show*, Channel Ten.

Peck, M.S., Dr., *The Road Less Travelled*, U.K., Simon & Schuster Ltd., 1984.

Prejean, Helen, Sr., *Dead Man Walking*, St. Joseph of Medailles, New Orleans, 1993.

Courses: *Marriage Enrichment Seminar, Counselling, Boundaries* and *Relationships, Family of Origin, Healthy Family, Dysfunctional Family*, Handouts, Burswood, 2001.

EVIDENCE

EXHIBIT ONE

19

25/2/02

DC Audio
fifty dollars

loan

50 —

J Meade

22

22/4

DC Audio
100 —

100 —

J Meade

EXHIBIT TWO

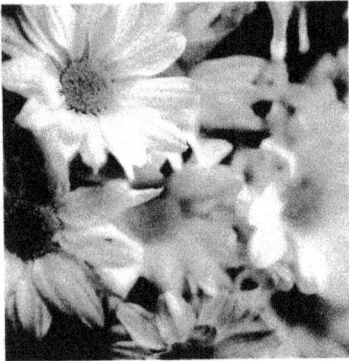

Dear Mum,

THANK YOU SOoo
Much for everything
you've done for us.
We're forever
Grateful.
Love Always
Jaung
&
Luke

P.S. This was ~~Luke's~~ idea.

Presented to

Elizabeth (Muffins)

By

Dale Meade with love

On

Our reconciliation 2002

7pm. Friday July 30th 2004

in our 4 years separation

2 years back with Beth

She is much better than when you threw her out
at 16 years old out of Aspern ~

You are beautiful, bubbly, lovable

No more coupons from me

Get healthy like an eagle, they ye find another eagle.
without a meal/them. Tell Giacq & Joan if was me changing
the money to be paid back. It was, when I get manic, I
like to settle old scores, I don't know my boundaries ~
When diagnosed we could have divorced, I did not need to
try & kill myself!

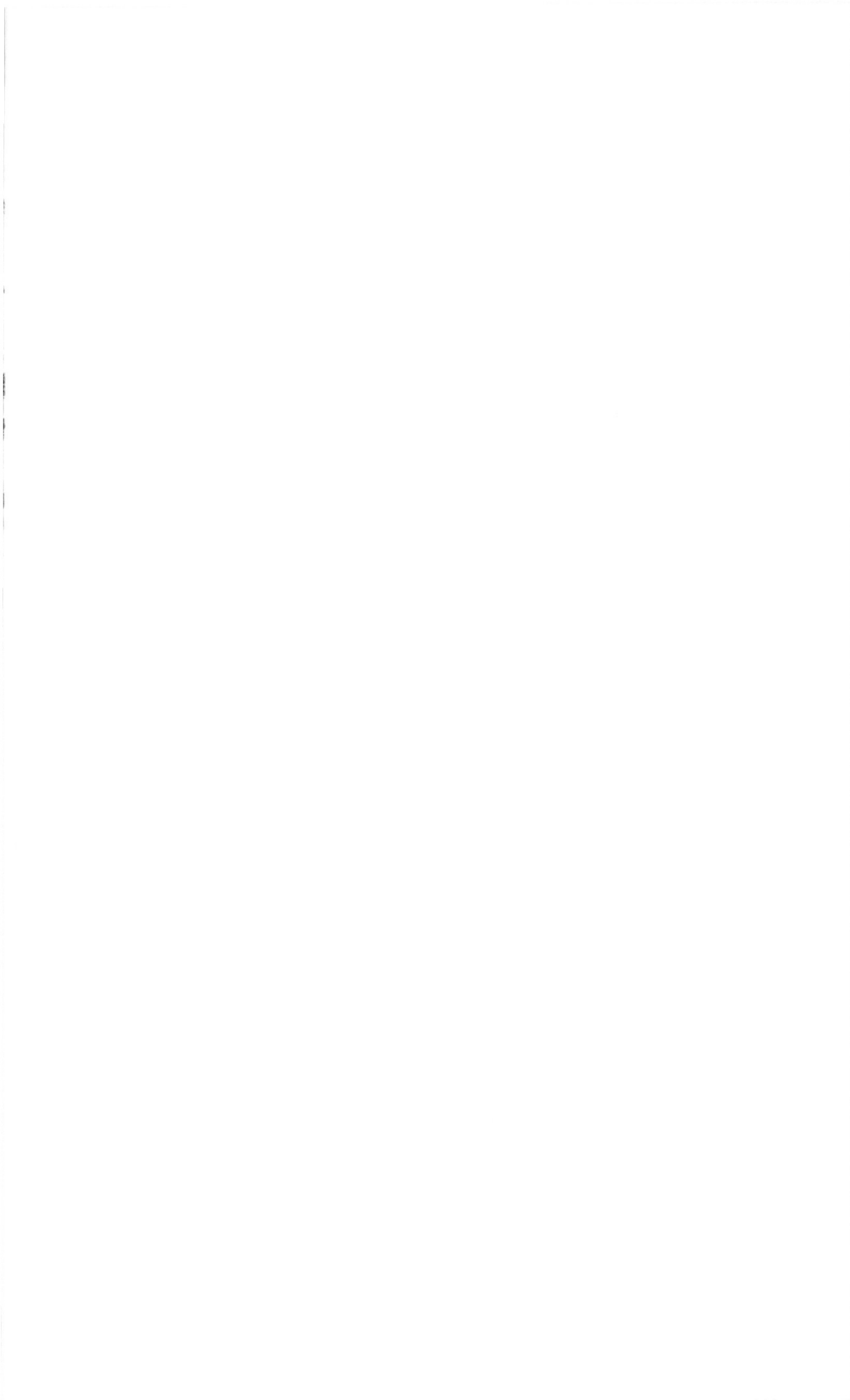